The Integrated Practitioner

Surviving and Thriving in Health Practice

BOOK 1 OF *THE INTEGRATED PRACTITIONER* SERIES

JUSTIN AMERY

Radcliffe Publishing
London • New York

Radcliffe Publishing Ltd
St Mark's House
Shepherdess Walk
London N1 7LH
United Kingdom

www.radcliffehealth.com

British Library Cataloguing in Publication Data

A catalogue record for this book is available from the British Library.

ISBN-13: 978 184619 772 7
Volume set ISBN-13: 978 184619 950 9

The paper used for the text pages of this book is FSC® certified. FSC (The Forest Stewardship Council®) is an international network to promote responsible management of the world's forests.

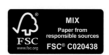

Typeset and designed by Darkriver Design, Auckland, New Zealand
Printed and bound by Hobbs the Printers, Totton, Hants, UK

Contents

These books are dedicated to my Dad, Tony Amery, who was a wonderful doctor and who is still my inspiration.

About the author

I am a full-time practising family practitioner and children's palliative care specialist doctor working in the UK. I have also spent some years working in Uganda and other sub-Saharan African countries.

I enjoy teaching, writing and mentoring. I am a medical student tutor at the University of Oxford, a trainer in general practice, and I have designed and set up children's palliative care courses for health professionals in the UK and Africa. I have worked with 'failing practices' to help them turn round; and also with health professionals who are struggling (as we all do from time to time).

I have always had an interest in philosophy and spirituality, and have studied this at postgraduate level. I have carried out some research into education and training of health professionals around the world and I continue to explore that interest.

I have previously written two books: *Children's Palliative Care in Africa* (Oxford: Oxford University Press, 2009) and the Association for Children's Palliative Care (ACT) *Handbook of Children's Palliative Care for GPs* (Bristol: ACT, 2011). I particularly enjoy reading and writing poetry.

At heart, though, I am a practitioner and a generalist. What is more, as you can probably see, I am rather a jack of all trades, and a master of none.

I have been motivated to write this book as I am hoping to explore practical ways of practising health that help us all, patients and practitioners alike, to become a little more healthy, and a little more whole.

Acknowledgements

These books have been brewing up over many years and so there have been very, very many influences upon them. There are far too many people to mention and thank without risking leaving someone out, so I shall just mention those who have been immediately involved.

Firstly, thank you to those very kind and patient people who helped review the drafts and gave such helpful feedback: Maria Ward, Penny Thompson, Meriel Lynch, Tom Nicholson-Lailey, Peter Burke, Penny Moore, Susan McCrae, Caitlin Chasser, Louise Rutter, Polly Steele, Rachel Samson, Laura Ingle and Maddy Podichetty.

I would also particularly like to mention Chris Smith, who not only gave very useful feedback on these books, but who also helped me to develop a lot of the ideas in them through his leadership of the Oxford Advanced Consultation Skills Course that I help him with, and over a few pints in the pub as well.

Thanks as well to Gillian Nineham of Radcliffe Publishing, who was brave (or daft) enough to put her faith in these rather unconventional offerings; suggest numerous areas for improvement and offer tremendous support and encouragement in their publication. Thanks also to Jamie Etherington and Camille Lowe for all their help in putting them together.

I would like to thank my colleagues at Bury Knowle Health Centre in Oxford, Helen House Hospice in Oxford, Hospice Africa in Kampala, Uganda, and Keech Hospice in Luton. They have all shown utmost patience and perseverance as I have led them on various merry dances, contortions and deviations in the name of 'good ideas', rarely reminding me of the 99% which failed, and always supportive of the 1% that, miraculously, did.

Of course I can't forget Karen Bateman (the doctor) and Karen Amery (the missus) who has been a continuous and never-ending source of sound advice, support and wisdom.

Finally, I would like to offer a huge thank you to Polly who, on a cliff top in Spain, gave me the courage to risk writing this stuff down and making it public.

Introduction to the series

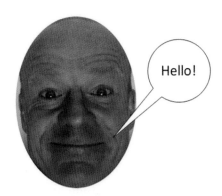

Hello!

Hello and welcome! This is me. You and I will be sharing a journey through this book, so you may wish to know what I look like. Because practice can't happen without practitioners, I will be popping up now and again, to test-drive some of the ideas that we will be discussing.

WHY ARE THESE WORKBOOKS NEEDED?

If you are, like me, a modern-day practitioner, you are probably still dedicated to the idea of good practice, but feeling rather buffeted by many and various winds of change that are sweeping through. You are also probably feeling (like me) that it would be good to have two minutes to sit back and reflect a little: to think about what's working and what's not; and maybe even to find a little balance.

If this is how you feel, you have come to the right place. So welcome!

In this series of workbooks we will be doing exactly that, taking a little time out, thinking about what we are doing, looking at things from different perspectives and using different lenses, and trying out some practical ways of making our practice more effective, more efficient, and (above all) more satisfying.

On the other hand . . .

If you are, like me, a modern-day practitioner, you will probably also be moving far too quickly to have any time for doing anything except what you need to be doing. In other words, you probably don't feel you have time for luxuries like sitting back and thinking. Frustrating though it may be, you probably have time to do only what you *have* to do, rather than what you *want* to do.

If this is how you feel, you are still in the right place, so welcome again!

In this series of workbooks, we will be working under the clock, recognising that there are boxes to tick and targets to hit. No doubt you don't just need to keep up to date, you need to prove you are keeping up to date too, for appraisal, or for review, or for revalidation. So, as we go along, we will be providing practical examples that will help you not just to reflect upon but actually to develop your practice.

What's more, we will even be providing appraisal certificates, so our appraisers, line managers and bosses will stay happy too!

But you're gonna have to serve somebody, yes indeed
You're gonna have to serve somebody,
Well, it may be the devil or it may be the Lord
But you're gonna have to serve somebody.

– Bob Dylan

WHY DID I WRITE THEM?

I have written these workbooks because there doesn't seem to be anything out there that scratches my itch. Our experience of real-life health practice is messy, complex and often chaotic. It doesn't seem to bear much resemblance to the practice we read about, or even the practice we try to teach our students and trainees.

Modern scientific and philosophical understandings of the universe are complex, messy and relational too. But our models of health and health practice often seem to be built on glib and simplistic models, or they fall into dualistic discussions (for example, about 'patient-centred' or 'practitioner-centred' care; or about 'traditional' or 'alternative' practice; or even about 'disease' and 'health'). Is the world really like that?

I have also written these books as I am worried about the levels of demoralisation and burnout among students, trainees and colleagues that I meet, right across the globe. Of course we can all get a bit tired, burnt out, and maybe even ill. If we are honest, we are often sceptical and occasionally a little cynical about what we do. But if we are even more honest than that, at heart we believe in what we do, because we think it is important.

It's not that we want to turn the clock back. We can feel a considerable (if quiet) sense of pride in how far health practice has developed. But perhaps we'd also like to think that, in the 21st century, there is a way for our practice to include and yet somehow to transcend what has gone before. It's not that we want to reject the practicalities, the science, the technology and the politics. On the contrary, I think most of us wish to accept and value them. But we also want to do what evolution always does: including, building upon and then transcending what has gone before. In so doing, maybe we can also rediscover the art of what we do, and perhaps even find a way of expressing ourselves with a little more poetry.

WHAT WILL BE IN THEM?

The answer to that is simple really. We are hoping to look at practice from different perspectives, and using different lenses, so each book takes a different view.

- Workbook 1 – *Surviving and Thriving in Health Practice*. We are the foundation of everything we do. Without us there would be no health practice. We are our own most useful tools. So, in the first book, we will look at how we can keep ourselves sharp, surviving and thriving in practice.
- Workbook 2 – *Co-creating in Health Practice*. As practitioners, whenever we come into contact with our patients, we create something very familiar but also very strange: a relationship. This relationship is neither me nor the patient, but some sort of third entity, which has an existence of its own, partly from me, and partly from the patient. This 'co-creation' is arguably our most powerful tool, but it is a tricky one to use. So we will focus on that in the second workbook, considering how we might practise in a way that co-creates healthier and happier existences, for both our patients and ourselves.
- Workbook 3 – *Turning Tyrants into Tools in Health Practice*. As practitioners we have a vast array of tools that we can use: time, computers, money, information, colleagues, equipment, targets, our workplaces and so on. If they get out of balance, however, each of these tools can become a tyrant, so that it has control of us, rather than the other way round. So in workbook 3 we will be looking at some of the most important tools (and tyrants), considering how we can stay in control of them (and not vice versa).
- Workbook 4 – *Integrating Everything*. Health practice is, ultimately, a single integrated thing. While workbooks 1–3 have been looking at the different 'bits' of this 'whole', workbook 4 is where the rubber hits the road, because it is here that we try to put it all together and come up with ways that we can integrate everything into a happier, healthier and more skilful whole within the real-life, complex and messy world of health practice.
- Workbook 5 – *Food for Thought*. We are practitioners, so we are practical, and interested in practice. So we will leave the theory until last. But most of us like a little bit of theoretical background to give context to, and to underpin our practice.[1] So workbook 5 tries to provide that. Everything that exists does so against a background. Indeed the word 'exist' means to 'stand out'. All of our experiences, beliefs and understandings of health practice derive from a living, organic and constantly moving context: whether scientific, philosophical, cultural, aesthetic, biological or spiritual. It is useful therefore to spend a little time understanding and reflecting on these building blocks of who we are. As practitioners, we don't always have time to do this, so we will leave this book until last. It will be a little luxury for those with a little more time, not essential, but hopefully a bit nourishing. Like a fireside cup of cocoa.

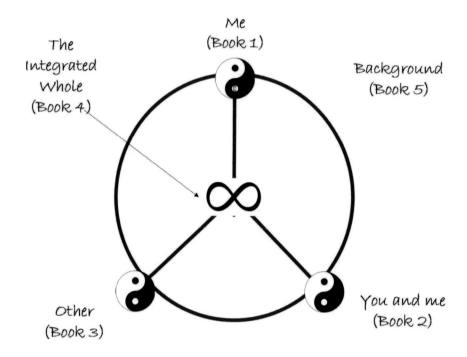

The
Integrated
Whole
(Book 4)

Me
(Book 1)

Background
(Book 5)

Other
(Book 3)

You and me
(Book 2)

WHAT PERSPECTIVES AND APPROACHES WILL THEY USE?

In the 21st century we practise healthcare in a strange tension.

Science has taught us that we live in a highly relational, messy, multidimensional, complex, blurry and even chaotic universe. The humanities and philosophy have taught us that much of what we hold to be 'true' is relational and cultural and socially constructed. The arts teach us the value of creativity and expression in all walks of life. Spirituality teaches us about perspective, the value of awareness, and the fundamental interconnectedness of all things.

However, despite this relationality, creativity and complexity, we seem to be practising in a world that seems ever more bound and codified, with ever more targets and tick boxes, according to models that seem unrealistically geometric and two-dimensional, and with ever less room to breathe and to express ourselves.

So, in these workbooks, we will try to be practical and pragmatic. While we may not necessarily like the rules, regulations, guidelines, laws and targets that have nosed into our practice, we recognise that they have their uses. We know that health is a political football, and we are used to being kicked around a bit.

As practitioners in the 21st century we also value (and sometimes worry about) the advances that science and technology have brought. As practitioners, we are scientists, and we have a duty to do our best to ensure that what we do is as safe and effective as possible. We recognise that finding an evidence base for what we do is important not just for safety, but for development too.

So in these workbooks, we will start from the premise that we should, wherever possible, look for empirical evidence for what we are suggesting. On the other hand, we will remain vigilant to the blind spots of the empirical and technological approach, and look for alternatives to fill any gaps that we find.

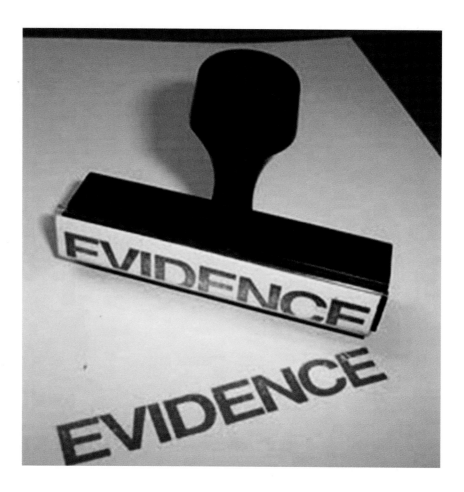

Wherever possible we will look for empirical evidence for what we are suggesting.

As modern practitioners we are scientists, and also technicians, but we are artists too. There is an art to being a practitioner, and in fact practice is an art. We might lose sight of it sometimes, but we are in the business (and busy-ness) of trying to create healthier and happier existences for our patients, and hopefully for ourselves too.

So in these workbooks we will be using plenty of imagery, art and illustration to engage the more creative sides of our brains, and to remind us that integrated practitioners need to be able to find balance between creative and practical.

These days, we don't tend to talk much about spirituality. Many of us would not think of ourselves as 'religious', and some of us might be horrified at the idea that modern-day practice should have anything to do with spirituality.

But most of us perhaps like to feel that there is some purpose or meaning behind what we do. We may hope that our practice connects with and somehow reflects the values and traditions of our families as well as of our broader societies and cultures. We deal with life and death, and so with the many existential and spiritual questions that arise as a consequence. If we are to be integrated practitioners, we need to have a handle on these too.

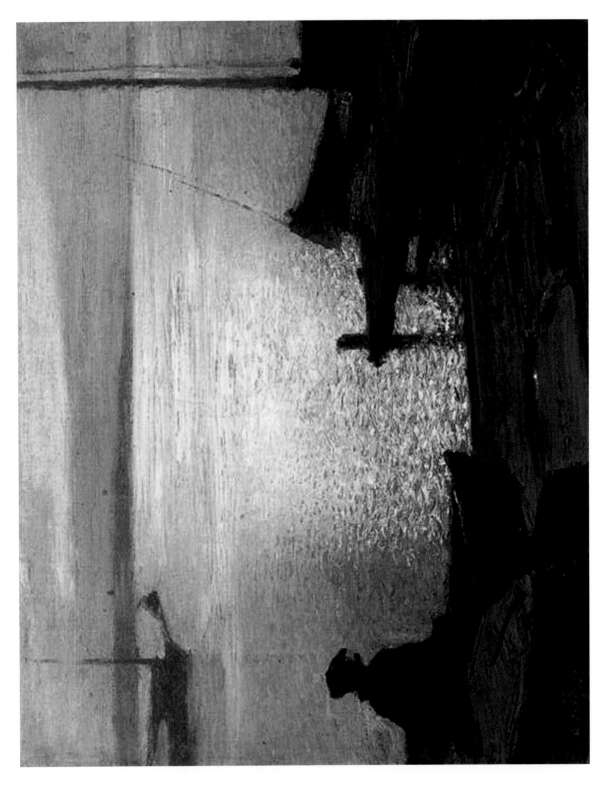

'*Along the Mystic River*' – for some reason I have found myself drawn to rivers as I have written this book, so a few will be popping up as we go along.[2]

So, in these workbooks we will try to look around the edges and to peer through the gaps, asking not just: 'What should we do?' but also 'Why should we do it?' and 'What does it all mean anyway?'

Finally, we don't have to practise long to realise that there are some things that make no sense, and from which no sense can be made. Random and chaotic events, reactions and emotions may arise, surprisingly. These can be both deeply troubling but also deeply wonderful, in that they can give expression to the inexpressible. We practitioners are practical people. We like to 'do' things. But sometimes there is nothing we can do, because there is nothing to be done. At these times, we have to just 'be'. For just 'being', for making sense of nonsense, and for making nonsense of sense, there is nothing better than poetry. So we will be seeing a fair bit of that too.

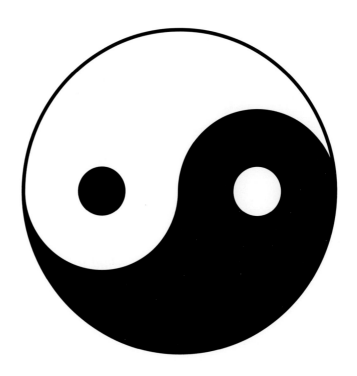

Symbols and rituals are fascinating things that in some way speak to us at a 'level beyond'. It is not often easy to make sense of them, and yet we may be surprised to find that our practice is full of them.

Ars Poetica

A poem should be palpable and mute
As a globed fruit,
Dumb
As old medallions to the thumb,
Silent as the sleeve-worn stone
Of casement ledges where the moss has grow –
A poem should be wordless
As the flight of birds.
*

A poem should be motionless in time
As the moon climbs,
Leaving, as the moon releases
Twig by twig the night-entangled trees,
Leaving, as the moon behind the winter leaves.
Memory by memory the mind–
A poem should be motionless in time
As the moon climbs.
*

A poem should be equal to:
Not true.
For all the history of grief
An empty doorway and a maple leaf.
For love
The leaning grasses and two lights above the sea–
A poem should not mean
But be.

– Archibald MacLeish[3]

POINTS AND PRIZES: SOMETHING FOR NOTHING

In the initial stages of this book, my publisher explained that medical publishing is at a turning point. Whereas before practitioners might choose a book that they would enjoy reading, nowadays they are too busy for that. So the upshot is that we only read books we need to read, rather than those we want to read.

A bit like Nanny McPhee...

The good news about adopting an integrated approach is we don't need to judge, we just need to adapt. If that is the way of the world, so be it, and so we have.

The particular way of the current world of health practice (at least where I currently work in the UK) appears to be a focus on objectives, outcomes, points and prizes. So the initial book has been adapted to match. Each chapter will contain activities and reflections that will meet common curriculum areas for medical and nursing practice. At the end of each book is a link to the Radcliffe Continuing Professional Development site, www.radcliffehealth.com/cpd, where you can download certificates that you can use for your CPD, appraisal or revalidation requirements.

OK, I admit it's a bit tongue in cheek, but there's no rule to say that we can't have fun while toeing the line, is there?

PROVISOS

I am, at heart, a practitioner, and a general practitioner at that. That means I am a bit of a jack of all trades, but master of none. I am partial, biased and subjective. The book is intended for all health practitioners but, inevitably, and despite my best efforts, no doubt the 'male', 'medical' and 'Western' nature of my experiences and thoughts will peep through. I hope you feel able to forgive them and look past them.

Also, I can quite honestly say that there is nothing new in this book, and I doubt there is anything in it that you could not find better argued and more coherently evidenced in other places. There is some philosophy, science, spirituality, art and poetry, but I am not a philosopher, scientist, guru, artist or poet. I am a health practitioner who dabbles.

So I have referenced those sources I can remember and can find. Others may be lost in the mists. But I do not claim any of the basic ideas in this book as my own. I have simply looked at them from my personal perspective and tried to put them together in a way that I have found useful in my own practice and in my own teaching. I hope you can enjoy them, and that you will forgive the numerous mistakes and omissions that you will undoubtedly find.

Chapter 1
'Me'

Case study (30 minutes)

Remember a really difficult episode from your health practice. What was it about? Who was involved? What happened? Really try to visualise yourself back there so that you begin to re-experience the reality of it.

Deep breaths...

Once your heart rate has come back down, your chest has loosened and your jaw has unclenched, write down all of the factors that made that day so bad. But write them under three headings, as follows.
1. 'Me' factors: all of the things about you on that day that might have contributed to your experience of the day.
2. 'We' factors: all the things about your relationships with patients and with colleagues that might have contributed to your experience of the day.
3. 'Other' factors: all of the other pressures constraints and external factors that might have been playing on your mind or influencing your experience of the day.

THE CRUCIAL IMPORTANCE OF ME

We talk about 'patient-centred care', or 'evidence-based care', or 'outcome-driven care' and so on. In integrated practice these are very important. We want to put our patients in the centre of our focus, we want to practise in a way that is properly founded in evidence, and we want to achieve healthy outcomes.

But the risk of terms like these is that they can distort and distract us from the reality of health practice which is always 'me-centred'. It may sound faintly heretical to suggest it, but **in health practice the most important person is the 'me'.**

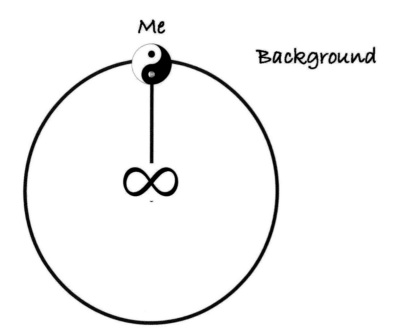

It seems strange to think that we are in relationship with ourselves. But that 'me' relationship is the foundation of our whole practice.

It is within me and through me that the universe expresses itself, and it is within and through me that I express myself to the universe.

Taken alone, I am nothing. I can only exist in relationship to something or someone else. I cannot conceive of existing outside the universe, or outside of relationship to other living beings.

Without me, the universe is just the interplay of forces, energy and matter. I 'create' the universe by being conscious of it, and in so doing I create the richness, depth and quality of what it is not just to exist but to live.

In the same way, without 'me', there is no health practice. It is always 'me' that offers help to those who feel unwell. When that 'me' is trained and qualified to help other 'me's' that are unwell, he or she is a professional health practitioner. There are many ways of defining health, many ways of seeking health, and many ways of offering healthcare, but none of these can happen without 'me'.

PLATE SPINNING AND THE PLATE BEING SPUN

Do you ever feel you are constantly spinning plates in your practice? Do you often feel you are constantly on (or over) the edge of balance and that all the plates might come spinning down? Worse still, do you sometimes feel as if *you are* the plate, constantly spinning and being spun by a universe of demands, obligations and targets? If so, read on.

We are constantly in relationship with other people, such as our patients, but also our colleagues, bosses, juniors, staff and so on. We are also always aware of a multitude of different factors and issues that may influence our practice (such as money, resources, environment, regulations, laws, ethics and so on). Each of these people, relationships and entities is like another plate that needs to be kept balancing and spinning if our 'performance' is to be effective.

As practitioners, we really are both plate-spinners and plates being spun, at one and the same time. That sounds quite unpleasant, but there is some good news, which is that at the centre of everything that spins is stillness and balance.

Activity 1.1: 30 minutes

Sit comfortably in your chair. Relax your jaw, neck, shoulders and tummy. Breathe deeply all the way in and slowly out.

Look at the image below. Where are your eyes drawn to?

Look slightly to one side. What happens to the wheel and how does it make you feel?

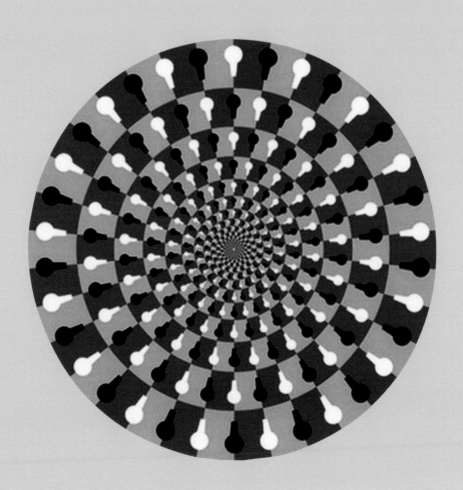

> When you feel like you are spinning, giddy and disorientated, reflect on the fact that your consciousness can create different realities and experiences by using different perspectives.
>
> Consider your perspectives. In practice, how do you see yourself? Is that perspective healthy or unhealthy?
>
> Allow your gaze to work its way round and round the wheel into the centre.
>
> Reflect on the fact that there is one place in a spinning wheel that is still. Where is it? Where is yours? How can you find that centre in your practice when everything around you is spinning?

WHY IS THE 'ME' SO IMPORTANT?

If we start to feel like this, if our practice seems to have too much spinning and wobbling, and not enough balancing and centring, it may be worth looking at the three fundamental relationships of practice again.

There is one person that is central to all of them. That is 'me'. However, it is often the 'me' that comes last.

That's topsy-turvy, and we can't spin plates, be plates being spun, and be topsy-turvy all at the same time. Without me, there is no 'we'. And without me, there is no one who can observe and use the 'other'. In short, without me, there is no practice.

The person that is both the subject and the object of that balancing is 'me', so I always have to start and end with 'myself' when practising healthcare in an integrated way.

In most health-related textbooks, books on communication, scientific literature and healthcare curricula we find that the focus is usually on 'you' (the patient) or 'other' things, like knowledge, competencies, science, organisation, regulations, targets, finances, ethics and so on and so on.

Curricula and assessments are very important and very useful. They help us (and others) know when we have achieved a certain 'bottom line' which we need in order to be able to practise proficiently and legally. However, they can have the unintended effect that, when we are taught, we are not taught in an integrated way, so that we focus only on one thing, or one group of things, rather than on the whole integrated process.

KEEPING OURSELVES HEALTHY

That is not to say that the 'me' can't also become too influential, or even tyrannical. If we practise selfishly, for our own ends rather that for the ends of the whole system, our practice may become unbalanced and ineffective. But it does mean we need to keep ourselves healthy if we are to have any hope of keeping our practice healthy too.

Often we lose sight of ourselves in offering healthcare. We can focus too much on the needs of the patient; or the approval of our peers or teachers; or on the targets we must hit; or of the money we spend and earn.

When we lose sight of ourselves we lose balance, and balance is at the heart of health. If we are not balanced, we cannot help our patients to become balanced.

As health practitioners we are the tools we use to practise our profession. A carpenter keeps his tools sharp. So to be effective tools for ourselves and our patients, we should aim to care for ourselves as skilfully and effectively as we care for our patients. We therefore have three strong, practical reasons to care for ourselves:

- to be compassionate to ourselves (we are as deserving as anyone else)
- to be compassionate to our patients
- to be compassionate to our colleagues, health systems and health processes.

Activity 1.2: 30 minutes

Read the poem by Daikaku on the following page.

What does it suggest about the reality of our experience and the creativity of our consciousness?

What are the potential limits of ourselves, and of our practice?

What is our practice based upon and built from?

How well do we take care of ourselves and our patients?

Whether you are going or staying or sitting or lying down

Whether you are going or staying or sitting or lying down,
the whole world is your own self.
You must find out
whether the mountains, rivers, grass, and forests
exist in your own mind or exist outside it.
Analyse the ten thousand things,
dissect them minutely,
and when you take this to the limit
you will come to the limitless,
when you search into it you come to the end of search,
where thinking goes no further and distinctions vanish.
When you smash the citadel of doubt,
then the Buddha is simply yourself.

– Daikaku

Chapter 2
Seeking happiness in our practice

Activity 2.1: 30 minutes

Find somewhere comfortable and allow your mind to settle.

Take yourself back to the day that you finally qualified. Try to remember how the future looked to you then. What did you expect and hope for from your career?

Did you feature yourself as a possible beneficiary of that career? Did you expect or hope that your career would make you happy? If so, why and how did you think it might make you happy?

Now come back to today. How has your career lived up to those hopes and expectations? In what ways does your career still make you happy? In what ways does it fail to make you happy?

Come back into the moment. Can you feel thankful for those ways it has made you happy? Can you try to change those things that make you unhappy?

Most of us would like to be happy in our work, and few of us would argue that being happier would not make us more effective. Of course we cannot be happy all the time, particularly because we often deal with people and situations which are very upsetting.

However, it is not too much to think that our job should be a source of happiness and pleasure overall.

Wishing to be happy in our work is not a self-centred aim. It is a compassionate aim, for if we do not value ourselves enough, our practice will become unbalanced, and we will start to fail both our patients and our wider responsibilities. So in caring for ourselves we are compassionate to ourselves, compassionate to those we care for, and compassionate to the whole system of health practice.

Perhaps we should therefore seek our own health and happiness as thoroughly and systematically as we seek the health and happiness of our patients and colleagues? It's an interesting if slightly sacrilegious thought, isn't it?

They all attain perfection when they find joy in their work.

– Bhagavad-Gita 18.45

LEARNING FROM THE EVIDENCE

As happiness is such a personal, subjective and relational concept, it defies easy definition or description. We know it when we have it, but we often don't fully understand why we are happy (or unhappy), still less what the 'right way' is to make ourselves feel happy.[4]

However, there is some useful evidence and experience. People have been studying and practising the pursuit of happiness, and in fact many of the world's oldest texts consider the question in great depth,[5] while researchers are using modern methods to study it right now.[6] These mystics, philosophers, scientists and psychologists do not agree on everything, but taken together some common themes emerge. Recent psychological and economic evidence[7] suggests that happiness seems to be related to:

- taking and keeping a balanced perspective
- having a sense of meaning and purpose
- meeting the basic needs of our loved ones and ourselves
- trying to be aware of, and stay in, the present
- dedicating ourselves to some challenge – not too much and not too little
- forming compassionate, generous and loving relationships with others
- being compassionate with ourselves
- creating a compassionate and integrated relationship with everything, through living what we believe to be a 'good life'.

Activity 2.2: 30 minutes

Try to grab a few moments of quietness.

Look at the diagram below in Image 2. Reflect on whether and how your job helps you to do what's in the five bubbles: connecting with others, being active, taking notice of the present, learning and teaching, and giving to others.

Then let your thoughts find their way to the middle bubble: your functioning. Out of 10, how would you rate your current level of functioning at work?

Finally, start to emerge out of the bubble and reflect deeply on yourself. How is your sense of well-being now? What levels of mental capital do you currently possess? Are these two things balanced in your life?

Come back to now. How are you feeling: better or worse?

Try to capture in your mind all the ways that your job is helping you to build your sense of well-being and mental capital. Perhaps also realise that there are some quite practical and do-able ways that you can become stronger in facing those things that may make you unhappy in your practice.

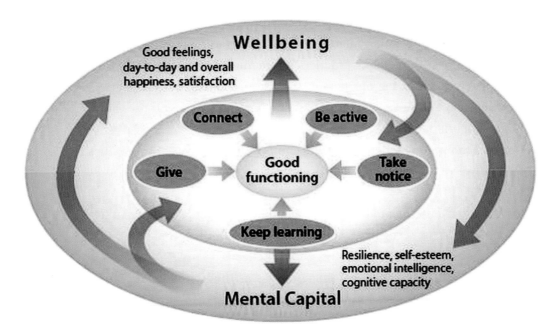

Happiness (usually referred to as 'well-being' in the scientific literature) is nicely presented here as in constant relationship with 'mental capital'. Some factors that seem to be important are also represented[8]

LEARNING FROM THE MASTERS

Be content with what you have; rejoice in the way things are. When you realise there is nothing lacking, the whole world belongs to you.

— Lao Tzu

The study of happiness is by no means new.

Buddhists have been systematically analysing, teaching and practising the pursuit of happiness for over two and a half thousand years. It is probably not surprising that they have a teaching about happiness which captures much of what modern evidence (as presented above) suggests. This is the so-called 'eightfold path'.[9]

> I myself am not a Buddhist, so I have no axe to grind, and I hope not to generate any antipathy if people have different beliefs and understandings about existence. In this workbook I have included some religious and mystic texts, as well as scientific and philosophical ones, because I think they have something to offer all of us, whatever our beliefs. I hope that we will be prepared to put aside any differences we may feel in order to look for similarities and opportunities for discovery.

A SUGGESTED PATH (OF SORTS) TO HAPPINESS IN PRACTICE

Pulling together all of this learning and experience from all of these sources, there seem to be a number of themes that might be helpful to us as health practitioners as we try to seek happiness through our practice. These might include the following.

- Keeping perspective: clarifying our perspective, setting our basic perspectives about the reality and illusions of our existence, and being clear about those values that are most important to us.
- Dedication and commitment: dedicating and committing ourselves fully to values and goals that we value the most, so that we focus our effort on what is most important.
- Leading a 'good life': choosing to try to live a 'good life' that acts out those values that are important to us, recognising that happiness cannot be an aim in itself, but can only be the product of the life we choose to lead.
- Being mindfully aware[10] and focused: seeing things as they actually are, rather than being buffeted by worries, anxieties and ruminations. From there being completely aware of and focused on what is truly going on, both within us and around us, so that we unify and focus our energy and awareness, and in so doing maximise the energy we receive in return.

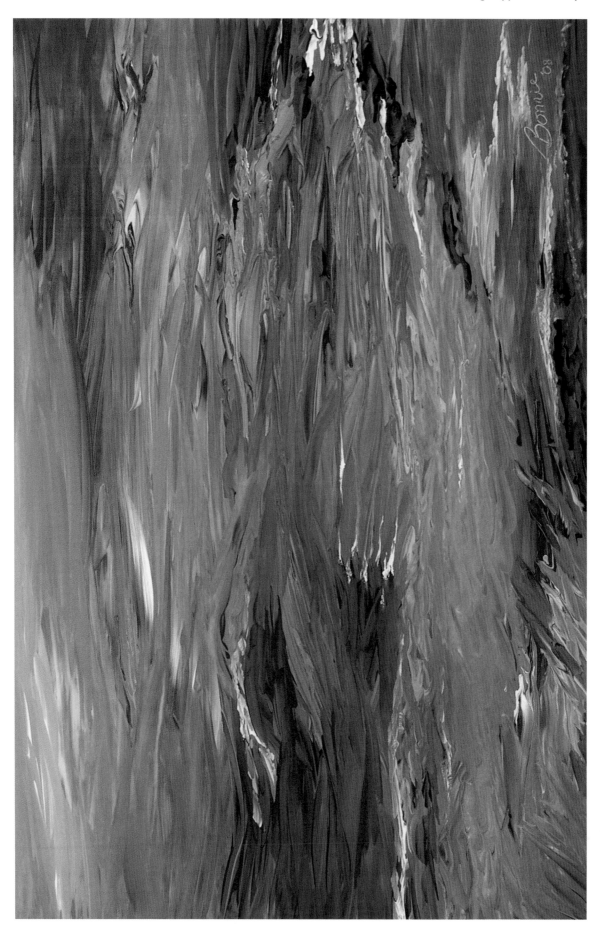

'Complete Happiness' – by Bonnie Lanzillotta[11]

- Communicating compassionately and skilfully: being in a continuous state of communication with ourselves and with others, and finding ways to communicate with ourselves and others in a way that is effective, compassionate, skilful and honest.
- Acting compassionately and skilfully: continuously trying to choose and act in ways that are skilful (by which we may mean more or less effective at caring) and which can help us to recognise the importance of continuous practice and continuous learning, so that our life becomes our learning and practice, and our learning and practice becomes our life.

HEALTH PRACTICE AS 'SELF-PRACTICE'

Being a health practitioner is a tremendous privilege, because it gives us the opportunity to do everything on this list. If we go about it skilfully, our work gives us the opportunity to meet our basic needs; to find and pursue something meaningful and purposeful; to form compassionate and loving relationships with our patients and others; to find perspective; to practise mindful awareness; and to live a 'good life' in which we can help others and build more harmony in life and in the universe. Fair enough, but how come so many practitioners are stressed and unhappy in their work?

Of course our work as health practitioners brings challenge. But a little challenge is a good thing, and an essential component of a good, happy life. On the other hand, too much challenge can unbalance us, leading to unhappiness and poor health. This is bad for us, bad for our patients and bad for the whole universal system.

Finding balance is easy. It just involves not falling over, which is a skill we learn early in life and which becomes an automated habit. Finding balance is also difficult, because it involves not falling over. The more we think about it and strive for it, the more we worry about falling. Striving simply creates another burden, which unbalances us more.

In the same way, the pursuit of happiness can be both easy and difficult. It is not something that is attainable by striving for it; but rather it is a side-effect of striving for other aims and purposes which are healthy for us and for others.[12]

There does not seem to be any intrinsic reason why health practice should not also be a source of deep happiness for each of us, even if it often doesn't feel that way. It would be good to explore whether our health practice can also be our 'self-practice', and that's what we would like to do in the rest of this workbook.

LEAVING ROOM FOR SCEPTICISM

Before we skip gaily off into happy-land, let's just take a sceptical moment. If you are, like me, an ageing practitioner with decades of practice under your belt, it may be hard not to scoff at what seems to be yet another load of mystical and meaningless 'coaching-speak'. These suggestions may seem too dreamy, impractical, irrelevant and idealistic to be of any use in the hurly-burly of modern health practice.

If so, I would ask you to consider that they might be rational. Happiness makes us work more efficiently and effectively, not less. The aim of this workbook is not to push or preach any one 'way' or another. It is simply to explore practical and pragmatic ways of practising that work, and that we can enjoy.

Of course my perspectives, like all perspectives, are limited, partial and biased. My knowledge claims, like all knowledge claims, are power claims and heavily tinted by my vanity.

So if you find that you are sceptical of what I am going to write, no doubt you are very wise. As practitioners we are aware of how easy it is to take advantage of the vulnerability of people when they are unwell. All knowledge claims need to be addressed with scepticism, and tested in practice, before they can be accepted.

But please read on, and judge for yourself.

Activity 2.3: 30 minutes

Reflect on the poem 'Happy the Man' below, or on the verse from the Bhagavad-Gita, or the saying from Lao Tzu written above. Consider how much your happiness is in your possession, and how much it is in the possession of others, or in the possession of the 'past', or in the possession of the 'future'.

Where it seems to be in the possession of past or future, remind yourself that science and philosophy show us that past and future are illusions born of our memory and of our imagination. Time does not flow. It just 'is', like space just 'is'.

How wise is it to invest our happiness in illusions?

Where your happiness seems to be in possession of others, whether people or things, reflect on the impermanence and fallibility of others. How wise is it to invest our happiness in impermanence and fallibility?

Come back to the present. Happiness is only ever felt in the present. Look around you and consider this. Can we be happy now? If not, what is stopping us?

Whether you feel you can be happy or not, consider those ways in which you may feel blessed, and resolve to start acting against those ways you may feel cursed.

Happy the Man

Happy the man, and happy he alone,
He who can call today his own:
He who, secure within, can say,
Tomorrow do thy worst, for I have lived today.
Be fair or foul or rain or shine
The joys I have possessed, in spite of fate, are mine.
Not Heaven itself upon the past has power,
But what has been, has been, and I have had my hour.

– John Dryden

Chapter 3

Clarifying our perspective

Activity 3.1: Finding nothing (30 minutes)

Sit comfortably but with a good posture.

Scan through your muscles, starting with the crown of your head, and working down through your face, throat, neck, shoulders, chest and arms, tummy, bottom, thighs, calves and eventually feet. With each out breath imagine tension flowing down and out through the soles of your feet, into the floor. You can do this quickly (within seconds), or slowly. It doesn't matter.

When you feel your tension has drained away, turn your attention inside to your thoughts and emotions. There are probably very many. Try and visualise them – give them form – maybe as clouds, or as shapes, or as colours. Don't engage with them but just watch them, as you would watch children in a playground. They may come up and nag you for your attention. If they do, kindly and gently reassure them and send them back.

After a little while, come to realise that there is a space between your thoughts. Start to notice the space more than the thoughts, and start to zoom in, so the space occupies more and more of your vision, and the thoughts gradually depart out of the periphery. Keep zooming in until all you can see is space.

Bring your attention back to how you are feeling and notice the peace and calm.

Welcome to nothing!

As we go about existing in this universe, we do our existing in the present moment. There is no other way we can exist.

If we want to experience our lives fully, rather than just existing within them, we experience this moment, then the next, then the next. We can imagine the future and remember the past, but we can only experience the present.

To experience the moment fully, we become aware of information from many sources: our senses, our memories, our emotions, our ideas, our thoughts, and our beliefs. Consciousness pulls all of these entities together to form one integrated experience of existence.

When we ex-ist (stand out) we exist against a background of non-existence. Just as our senses need black in order to be able to see white, so our minds seek the clarity of non-existence in order to be able to experience existence fully.

Therefore, before we can turn to the content and experience of existence as health practitioners, we might first wish to examine the background, without which we will have no context, and without which we can find no perspective.

THE ULTIMATE PERSPECTIVE – NOTHINGNESS

The background to everything is, by definition, nothing. 'Nothing' is such a strange concept that we may not give it much time. But unless we fully grasp that we have been created out of nothing, and will return to nothing, our life will be lived out of perspective and we may strive for useless or valueless things that will not lead to health or happiness.

Please note, we cannot say anything about the 'nothing', except that by definition it is nothing. But it is a nothing from which everything has sprung into ex-istence, by standing out against it. So the least we can say is that nothing has potential to generate something. We may therefore choose to name this nothing 'empty poten-tiality', but that is a question of belief. For some of us it may simply be the laws of the universe, for others it may be pure emptiness, for others it may be God. None of this is provable to anyone, as proof demands evidence, and evidence demands demonstration, and we cannot demonstrate nothing.

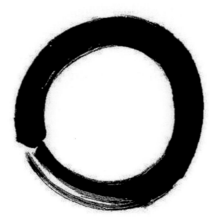

ULTIMATE BELIEFS

As health practitioners it does not much matter what we believe about the 'nothing'. Practitioners around the world have all views and none. But it does matter that we are aware of what we believe (and what we don't believe), because these are the beliefs that underpin our attitudes, ideas and ultimately behaviours, and it is those that will keep us grounded and the plates spinning.

Whatever we do or do not believe, we all have 'ultimate beliefs'. These are so-called because we cannot justify them. Ultimate beliefs are crucial, because they are the foundation for all our thoughts, choices and actions. As integrated practitioners, therefore, we may wish to try to become aware of, analyse and reject or restate our ultimate beliefs.

Activity 3.2: The ultimate beliefs game (30 minutes)

There are many ways we can try to become aware of our ultimate beliefs. Try this game with yourself. Take something you feel strongly about and ask yourself why. Notice that you have more than one 'self' and that these different selves can have a conversation. Keep asking yourselves why until you can't answer any more or until you loop back to the beginning. For example:

Self 1: What do we believe?
Self 2: We believe that euthanasia is wrong.

Self 1: Why?
Self 2: Because we believe that people should not kill other people.

Self 1: Why?
Self 2: Because we believe people's lives are valuable.

Self 1: Why?
Self 2: Because we believe within each person is part of a universal whole, and the universal whole is part of each person, and we do not want to damage the universal whole.

Self 1: Why?
Self 2: Because we believe without the universal whole there would be no cosmos and no life and no people.

Self 1: Why?

Self 2: Because we belief the universal whole is, in some way, continuously creative, and if we destroy parts of it, we are at risk of destroying the whole, which we believe would be wrong.

Self 1: Why?

Self 2: Because by damaging the whole, we would damage the individuals within the whole, and we believe that would be wrong.

Self 1: Why?

Self 2: Because we should not kill each other.

Self 1: Why?

Self 2: Oh, for God's sake. Can't we just get some peace and quiet?

Self 3: Who's God?

ULTIMATE PERSPECTIVES

Just as we have ultimate beliefs, we also have ultimate perspectives. These are the background and context to our lives. Often, in the busy-ness of health practice, we get so wrapped up with the next patient, or the next problem, that we lose track of 'what it's all about'. Without that background perspective, we lose perspective, and without perspective, as any artist will tell you, everything looks wonky.

Our perspective may be influenced by many things.[13]

- We may have different fundamental 'personality types'.
- Our perspectives may be affected by continuous and ongoing conscious and subconscious drives.
- We may be influenced by familial and cultural experiences, knowledge, understandings and approaches.
- We are 'wired' differently, so our brains may behave in different ways.
- We are subject to different environmental influences that may 'condition' us to behave in certain ways.

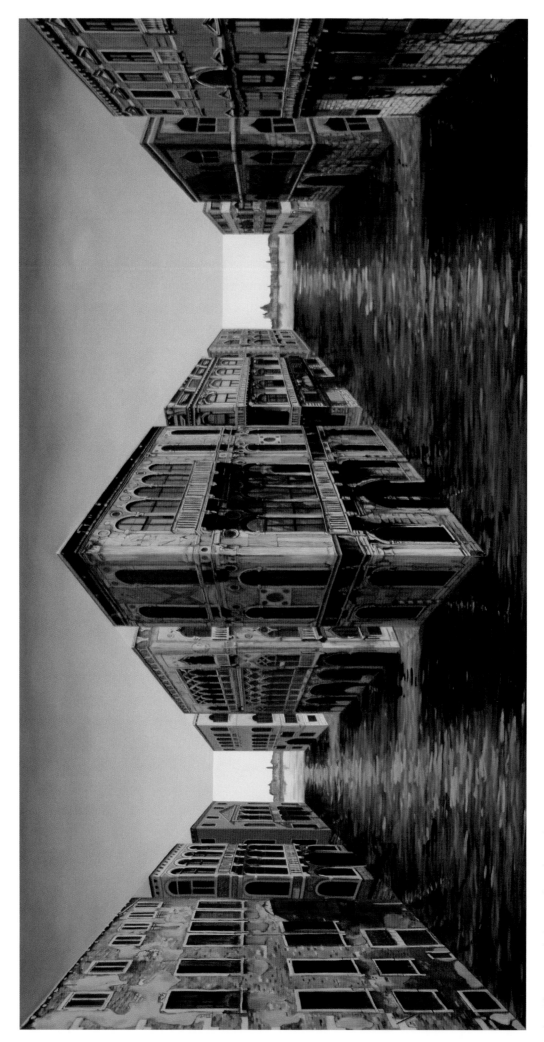

'Vanishing Venice' – by Patrick Hughes.[14] This painting is an interesting visual example of how, by taking different perspectives, we can see the same situations in entirely different light. Try focusing first on the buildings, and then on the spaces between the buildings, and see how the pictures seem to zoom in and out, towards you and away from you.

30

Activity 3.3: Your personality type (1 hour)

When thinking about our personalities, personality inventories can be helpful. While these tests can only ever be generalisations, they are often quite enlightening, and strengthening. If you can, try to take at least one or two tests,* and reflect on what you find out about yourself and your relationships with others.

A skilful practitioner is aware of his tools, and learns to work with his particular strengths and weaknesses. In the same way, a skilful practitioner may become more aware of her fundamental attitudes and perspectives, adapt those that need adapting wherever possible; and learn to work with those that are helpful, and to work around those that are unhelpful.

* *See* the endnotes for more information and directions for where to find some tests.[15]

As health practitioners, our personality types may be more likely to be perfectionist, self-critical or dependent than others.[16] These personality traits may mean that we place greater expectations on ourselves and colleagues, or believe that we should not make mistakes, or that illness is a weakness.

We might therefore find it useful to ask ourselves some difficult questions in order to get some perspective. Are we too self-critical? Do we tend to be perfectionist? Do we ever give ourselves a break and allow ourselves to be weak?

Activity 3.4: Fundamental perspective (30 minutes)

To become more aware of your own fundamental perspectives, perhaps you could try one of more of the following.

- Lie down and look up at the stars. Let your mind settle. After a while, look between the stars. Become absorbed into the emptiness. Stay a while, then, without becoming emotionally engaged, think of the last thing at work that really wound you up. Was it worth it?

- While we are on the subject of anger, what really makes you angry, even when you do have perspective? Anger is a tricky emotion to handle, but it is not always bad. It can give us energy to change the things we really believe need changing. What makes us angry, truly angry, is a good reflection of what is important to us. So, if you were a God, what's the first thing you would change to make the world a better place? Is your health practice taking the world closer to or further from your desired goal?

- Now imagine yourself on your deathbed, or write your own benediction. What would you look back on with pride and what would you consider to have been a complete waste of time and effort? Does your practice reflect that balance?

- Or, to finish with a more cheery one, imagine that you are given one wish by a fairy godmother. What would it be? Is your practice acting as the Fairy Godmother or as the Wicked Witch (locking you up in the tower)?

This Life, which seems so fair

This Life, which seems so fair,
Is like a bubble blown up in the air
By sporting children's breath,
Who chase it everywhere
And strive who can most motion it bequeath.
And though it sometimes seem of its own might
Like to an eye of gold to be fixed there,
And firm to hover in that empty height,
That only is because it is so light.
But in that pomp it doth not long appear;
For when 'tis most admired, in a thought,
Because it erst was nought, it turns to nought

— William Drummond

Chapter 4
Dedicating and committing

Activity 4.1: 30 minutes

Cast your mind back again to the day you first qualified. Then fast forward to today. You must have put in a huge amount of effort and time to get where you are. What made you do it? What were you aiming for? How did you find enough motivation to get here?

Cast your mind back to this morning. Has your professional life been successful in attaining what you originally dedicated yourself to?

How is your sense of commitment now? Is anything distracting you?

How are your energy levels? Would you say you are surviving and thriving, or would you say you are sinking and drowning?

DEDICATION AND COMMITMENT

Once we have worked out our personal perspective on things, it is a little easier for us to decide what to dedicate and commit ourselves to.

Dedication is the setting apart and proclaiming of something of significant importance, either to ourselves or to others. Commitment is the act of agreeing, with ourselves or with others, that we will focus on and target our efforts towards attainment of that value.

The power of a movement lies in the fact that it can indeed change the habits of people. This change is not the result of force but of dedication, of moral persuasion.

– Steve Biko

We can dedicate ourselves as a 'big thing' that we decide for the long term; but we can also commit ourselves for much smaller chunks of our existence: a year, a day, an hour, a moment. We tend to think of 'dedication' for 'big' things, and 'commitment' to the present and smaller things, but they can be used interchangeably.

VALUES

From day to day, or week to week, we may commit ourselves to a whole range of different things. Over the period of years, or indeed over our whole career, we might choose some more major aims, for example aiming for a certain position, or a certain income or a certain achievement.

However, positions and income and achievements can be illusory – seeming to have less value after attainment than when they were still a distant dream. So it can sometimes be more helpful to let positions and achievements look after themselves, and instead to commit ourselves to particular 'values'.

A value system[17] is a foundation upon which our deep choices, morals and ethics are based. If we try to live lives that meet our fundamental underlying values, we are more likely to feel more valuable and integrated. If we act in ways that go against our underlying values we feel split and less valuable.

It may therefore be helpful if we can become aware of those deep values that are most important to us, and to try to use those values to inform our choices, our thoughts, our speech and our actions. People tend to have different values, so this is a very personal choice. For example, we may wish to dedicate our practice to the pursuit of truth, or compassion, or knowledge, or justice or wisdom.

Activity 4.2: The values game (30 minutes)

Each of us has different values, but it is useful to try to work out which ones are most important to us individually. This is a little harder than it might seem. Often our values are so deeply hidden we have actually lost sight of them. But, just like ultimate beliefs, we all have them. To get to them, we can ask ourselves simple questions such as: 'What do I hope I will be remembered for when I am gone?'

Alternatively, we can play a little game with ourselves: the 'values game':

Self 6: Do we have any values?
Self 7: Of course we do! Who do you think we are?

Self 6: Sorry. I didn't mean to offend. What are they then?
Self 7: Er, well, we think that it's important to do the right thing.

Self 6: OK, but what do we mean by 'right'.
Self 7: Well, I suppose being compassionate perhaps, honest also, brave where possible, maybe just.

Self 6: OK, but are they all equal? Or do we feel some values are more valuable than others?
Self 7: How would I know?

Self 6: Well, set them in opposition and think which way we would choose. For example, if we were in a situation where telling the truth was not compassionate, which would we choose: to be a compassionate liar or a truthful brute?
Self 7: Hmm. I think we would prefer to be a compassionate liar.

Self 8: Speak for yourselves . . .

FIXING OUR DEDICATION

In the hurly-burly of health practice, we can easily get sucked into the demand of the next thing, and then the next thing. Without dedication and commitment our minds can wander, bad habits can knock us off course, and our energy can be dissipated without good effect.

This is particularly unhelpful for health practitioners as we have an awful lot to do, and little time within which to do it. We have to move swiftly, efficiently and effectively. If we are uncommitted to the moment; or if we do not feel dedicated to the task; we will be slower, inefficient and ineffective.

To try to counteract this, when we dedicate ourselves, it can be useful to try to 'fix' that dedication in our consciousness so that it becomes easy for us to access and remember. A helpful way to do this is to try to actually 'see' ourselves in our imagination, 'being' the future person we would like to become (whether in 10 years, 1 day or 1 minute).

When we imagine or visualise this, we can try to anchor that visualisation very firmly in our minds by developing a very rich and detailed picture. A cursory or fleeting picture tends to get lost very easily. By adding little details to the visualisation, and by building more texture and depth into it, we will anchor the dedication in our minds and give ourselves a better chance of expressing our core values in our practice.

> We often find we are stuck with automated behaviours which get triggered
> by certain situations, before we have a chance to intervene and stop them.
> For example, I have realised that if I am hungry and tired when I get home

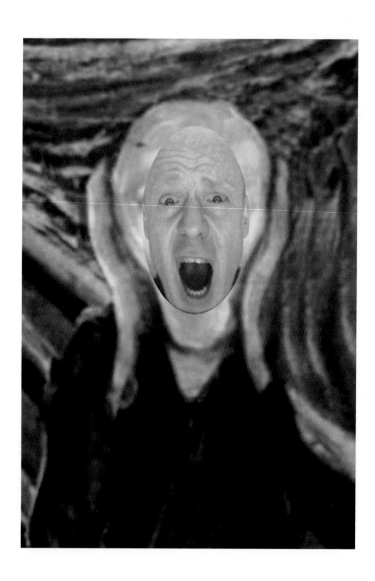

Peaceful dedication (my style) –
with apologies to Munch.

of an evening, and when I get in the kids are charging about being noisy (which is what kids always do just before bed when they are expecting a shouting father to appear any moment . . .) I almost always get grumpy or shout at them. I must have done this year in, year out, without stopping to ask myself why.

Recently I was reading about NLP techniques, and found an interesting article about how you can detect and behaviourally change these automated bad behaviours by clearly visualising an alternative outcome to the same situation. To fix these visualisations even more firmly, we can use visual or auditory reminders that we gradually train ourselves to automatically trigger the desired response. For example, I now have a place that I look at just above the front door, before I open it. Every time I reach the door I make myself look at it and experience a sense of calmness. Then I walk in.

I still shout, but not quite as much.

STRESS AND BURNOUT

In order to be able to dedicate and commit ourselves to our health practice, we hope to be able to clear our minds and to find perspective. If our minds and hands are already full, it is easy to lose sight of our values or to be swept into unskilful habits.

Most health practitioners are familiar with the sensation of feeling stressed. A little stress is a useful thing, as it increases our awareness and concentration. However, too much stress can lead us into over-engagement with our work; that in turn can lead us to 'burn out', which is a syndrome of under-engagement.[18]

Burnout reduces our productivity and saps our energy, leaving us feeling increasingly hopeless, powerless, cynical and resentful. The unhappiness burnout causes can eventually threaten our job, our relationships and our health.[19]

There are many factors that can influence levels of stress and burnout, and these are covered in the endnotes to this chapter.[20]

I have personal experience of burnout and ill-health. In 2001, I was at a 'high point' in my life. I was a partner in a good family practice in Oxford and medical director of a well-known children's hospice, I had just had my first research paper accepted for publication and I had set up and sold for a good price a company developing internet-based patient health records. At home we had just had twins (our third and fourth children). We had a lovely house. The money was good. Life was good.

A clean sheet

A clean sheet
A new start,
A blank canvas.

HA!

Etched, burnt, twisted, spent.

– JA

But it didn't feel good. I had the sense of going faster and faster, but going nowhere. My 'success' tasted bitter, not sweet. My dreams were full of dead and dying children from my hospice work and of my 'failure' to 'save' them. A pervasive sense of hopelessness and futility was overtaking me remorselessly, no matter how fast I ran, or how many new challenges I took on.

At a Christmas party one evening, the floor seemed to drop from beneath me. I went outside, started to cry, and didn't stop crying for several days. In that time, I experienced a deep and pure terror quite unlike anything I had known before or since. I felt I had lost all hold on reality, and that I was only holding by my fingertips to the edge of sanity, with the abyss yawning beneath me. It took me several months to come through that, and to this day (12 years later) I still occasionally get a deep sense of dread, hovering on the cusp of sheer panic (usually when I am about to start public speaking!). But I think I learnt more from those experiences of pure, primal terror than I have from the rest of my life put together.

If or when we think we might be burning out, our perspectives and values can be distorted, so it is wise to try to get objective evidence. It is not always easy for health practitioners to ask for help with our own health, so a useful first step can be to try completing a burnout inventory, like the one below.

Activity 4.3: The Burnout Inventory (20 minutes)

There are a number of tools available to help you get a more objective idea of whether you are a bit burnt out. The one below is copied from Mindtools* website, with their kind permission. Please go to the website and use it there because it helps them maintain the site, and also because it has a wealth of other useful resources (and no, I am not a shareholder . . .).

Question	Never	Rarely	Some-times	Often	Very Often
Do you feel run down and drained of physical or emotional energy?					
Do you find that you are prone to negative thinking about your job?					
Do you find that you are harder and less sympathetic with people than perhaps they deserve?					
Do you find yourself getting easily irritated by small problems, or by your co-workers and team?					
Do you feel misunderstood or unappreciated by your co-workers?					
Do you feel that you have no one to talk to?					
Do you feel that you are achieving less than you should?					
Do you feel under an unpleasant level of pressure to succeed?					
Do you feel that you are not getting what you want out of your job?					
Do you feel that you are in the wrong organisation or the wrong profession?					
Are you becoming frustrated with parts of your job?					
Do you feel that organisational politics or bureaucracy frustrate your ability to do a good job?					
Do you feel that there is more work to do than you practically have the ability to do?					
Do you feel that you do not have time to do many of the things that are important to doing a good quality job?					
Do you find that you do not have time to plan as much as you would like to?					
Total					

* For more information about how to score the inventory, as well as for more useful resources, go to: www.mindtools.com/stress/Brn/BurnoutSelfTest.htm

If you find you are burnt out, you are not alone, not by any means. Burning out is a sign of your compassion, so that is positive. Falling off your bike is just another step in learning to stay on it. Episodes of burnout can be times of great personal awareness, insight, learning and development. Burnout can lead rapidly to reignition if you care for yourself with the same compassion and skill with which you care for your patients.

Physician, heal thyself.

Which is easy to say, but very hard to do. Sometimes, when feeling like this, we feel alone and, what's more, we feel like we need to be alone. Asking for help, even from those we love, just seems like too much effort: worthless and pointless.

Let Me Be Alone
Oh let me be alone, far from the eyes and faces
Let me be alone, a while, even from you:
My soul is like a desert, sick of light filled spaces,
The urge of useless winds, the skies of pitiless blue:
Let me be alone, a while, in twilight places,
Waiting the merciful night, the stately stars
And the dew

— Sara Teasdale

But, even so, it may be wiser to do the simple and compassionate thing, and to ask for help anyway. Talking things through in detail will help us get a different perspective and see opportunities where before stood only insurmountable challenges. More importantly, it helps us realise we are not alone, that there are people who care, and that there is a worth to our lives and to ourselves.

If you feel like this, please read on, because in the next chapters we will be looking at ways to reignite and reintegrate ourselves.

RESILIENCE

All this talk of stress and burnout might give us the impression that we are drowning swimmers in a pool full of sharks. The fact that we have got this far, and that we are still going, should help us to realise that we are probably more resilient than we give ourselves credit for. The glass may be half full, not half empty.

In practice, each of us has an inbuilt buffer which helps us cope with stresses that are an inevitable part of daily life. This buffer is known as our resilience. When we are being put under pressure, we use a variety of coping strategies to help us defend our resilience. It is when our coping strategies become overwhelmed or weakened that we become vulnerable to stress and burnout.

There are a number of factors that contribute towards our resilience, the most important of which is having (and fostering) caring and supportive relationships. But there are many others, which centre on having insight into one's own strengths, weaknesses, emotions and drives; being realistic about what is achievable, but not being scared to have a go; and remembering to congratulate ourselves when small successes are won.

Activity 4.4: Build your resilience (30 minutes)

Have a look through the following suggestions for how to improve personal resilience, reflect on how you are doing, and choose one or two concrete things that you will change, this week.

- Eat well, sleep well, exercise and relax regularly.
- Have regular fun with family or friends, and make connections with them.
- Be optimistic: your mind will visualise what you fear, but it will also visualise what you want. Focus on the latter, not the former.
- Be realistic but positive about yourself: there are things that you can't and never will be able to do. Let them go. There are things you can do. Do them.
- Be decisive: once you have decided what you want to do, do it. Don't give up, detach, or delay in the hope something will turn up.
- Accept and embrace change: change brings loss, but also opportunity. If something didn't work, let it go, and look for the opportunity that has taken its place.
- Look on the bright side: painful things and failures happen, and we can't change that, but we can interpret these more or less positively. Everything that doesn't kill us has the potential to make us stronger.
- Keep moving: stay mindful of your values and goals, and try to make regular steps towards them, however small.
- Be a survivor, rather than a victim. You have got where you have got to, and you are still going, despite what happened.

- Look for self-discovery: whatever happens, good or bad, consider what it teaches you about yourself.
- Express yourself: your body will want to express itself, maybe through art, or sport, or socialising, or spirituality, or travel, or something else. Help it on its way by setting aside time and space to do so.

COMMITMENT AND DEDICATION IN HEALTH PRACTICE

In the crazy world of modern health practice, time is at a premium. Setting aside moments for dedication and commitment can seem like an idealistic, unachievable goal. But if we take a different perspective, perhaps we can see that it is not so much idealistic as an essential, professional duty. If we don't know where we are going, what our values are, or what we want to achieve, how can we provide focused and useful help to our patients within our day-to-day practice?

It does not have to be a big deal. For the major questions, such as 'what do I want to do with my life', perhaps we do need to allow a bit more time every year or so. For small things, though, it only takes a few seconds to fix our dedication, and so we can fit this easily into a working day.

> I run twice-daily (sometimes thrice-daily), very busy surgeries of around 20 consultations and then phone calls, visits and paperwork. I have found that I can go much more quickly and effectively if I arrive half an hour early, go through the notes, and literally imagine each patient, just for 5–10 seconds, trying to experience what life may look like from their perspective. Then, just before each patient comes in, I glance at a picture on my wall that I have 'anchored' to help me empty my head so that I can try to dedicate my entire energy and focus on the next patient.

The Vietnamese Zen teacher Thich Nhat Hanh made some suggestions for the actual practice of dedication and commitment as follows.

- Ask yourself, 'Are you sure?' This helps us to refocus our energies on what is valuable to us.
- Ask yourself, 'What am I doing?' This helps us settle distracted thinking and focus on the most effective and skilful actions.
- Be aware of your habits. By recognising and addressing automated 'bad habits', we have a better chance of staying committed and focused.
- Cultivate compassion. By practising compassion in our practice, we are better motivated to stay on the right path.

Ultimately, we have a choice. We always have a choice. Health practice can be draining: physically, mentally and spiritually. There is nothing more exhausting than trying to heal sick and damaged people. Health practice can also be restoring: physically, mentally and spiritually. There is nothing more rewarding than trying to heal sick and damaged people.

Day by day, moment by moment, we can veer between these extreme perspectives. If we look down, we may see an abyss. If we look up, we may see heaven. And if we look straight ahead, we may just find a bridge which will get us where we want to go. Dedication and commitment is about trusting that bridge and taking the first step, and then the next, and the next . . .

The World

The world, laid out
Breathtaking beauty
I stand, high, high above.
The breath of life rushing through me

Its joys unfathomed.
Unfathomable
I feel, deeply, deeply.
The joy of love pumping through me

And then, I look down

Down into an abyss
Dark and calling.
Still high above,
The terror numbing me

A bridge, stretching forward
Narrow, swaying.
To turn back or to run?
I run madly.
I run gladly.

– JA

Chapter 5
Practising righteously

Activity 5.1: How good are you? (30 minutes)

Many of us, maybe even most of us, consider that we aren't quite good enough. Our patients may not be too reassured if they knew that.

Even more worryingly, some of us consider that we are really good. These are the ones the patients should really be worried about.

Sit quietly for a second and ask yourself: how good am I?

Don't let yourself off until you have given yourself an answer. Perhaps even score how good you are as a percentage, with 0% absolutely, crushingly useless and 100% dreamily, wonderfully perfect.

Now think back to the fateful day when you were let loose on your first ever patient. Remember your stumbling, clumsy and perhaps even dangerous attempts. Now re-score yourself. How good are you?

Now think of the best colleague you know. Think of everything she does and compare yourself to her. Now re-score yourself again. How good are you?

Likely as not, you will now have three different scores. Why? Because value is subjective, and we have no clear and universal definition of what 'good' is.

If we don't know where we are starting from, how on earth do we know how to get wherever we want to go?

RIGHTEOUSNESS IN HEALTH PRACTICE

Our values act as a strong foundation for our actions, but there are other foundations too. In every country there are laws, in every religion there are rules, in every philosophy there are wisdoms, and in every profession there are guidelines and regulations.[21]

When we apply the whole process of living according to our deep values, we call that living 'righteously'. We may have drifted away from the use of that word, perhaps because sometimes it suggests self-righteous dogmatism: that we know better than others what is right and what is wrong.

But the original meaning of the word was not like that. The term righteous comes from the old English 'rihtwis', which is a combination of 'right' and 'wise'. Few of us would dispute that it is both right and wise to act out of our deep values, or wrong and unwise to act against them.

SPLITTING

If we act or speak in ways that are run counter to our deep values, it sets up a tension within us that leads to a process of splitting the 'way I am' from 'the way I want to be'. The more we split the less valuable we become in our own eyes.

It is hard to for us to be integrated practitioners when we split like this. On the other hand, in a messy, complex and relational universe, we always have the right to make mistakes, and we always have the chance to create a new present, whatever the past mistakes we have made.

If we become aware of past mistakes, which may have led to unrighteous actions or words, we always have the choice to make good those actions or words where we can, and admit our actions or words and ask for forgiveness where we cannot.

> And if we start to get down on ourselves, we always have the choice to laugh at the ridiculousness of our vanity, forgive ourselves and smile at our daftness.

It ain't what you do, it's the way that you do it.

– Melvin 'Sy' Oliver and James 'Trummy' Young

ACTING RIGHTEOUSLY IN HEALTH PRACTICE

In a relational universe, it is hard to maintain with any certainty that any one particular moral code or ethical framework is more or less righteous than another. However, if we turn things around a little, and focus on our motivations rather than our actions for a little while, things become simpler. If our actions are motivated by our deep values, for example if we act out of compassion, or honesty, then we unlikely to act un-righteously.

> We will come to looking at what 'righteous action' may mean in regard to patients later in the series. The focus of this workbook, however, is ourselves.

When we first start in practice, we have to go slowly, and our journey seems disjointed, stop–start and clunky as we keep being confronted by new choices and new options. In the face of the rapid-fire 'act-choose-act-choose-act-choose' of modern health practice, it can seem as though we have no time to be considering the righteousness of each and every choice or option. But in fact the opposite is true.

> A skilled practitioner can become aware of his or her perspective and values; and apply these mindfully and skilfully in the practice of health-care consistently and effectively as he or she goes along. This might seem counter-intuitive, but let's reflect for a second.

If we think about it, a great deal of what we do in practice originally took time and effort to acquire, and when we first started we were slow and awkward. However, a little later on these practices became so familiar as to be almost automated. A truly skilled practitioner operates at an intuitive level, known as a 'flow state', within which he or she acts almost automatically and yet stays constantly and mindfully aware of acting, at one and the same time (we will go into more detail about how we may achieve this is in later chapters and workbooks in this series).

> Think of a skilled surgeon operating, or a skilled diagnostician assessing, or a skilled therapist listening. They have become so masterful at what they do that they can allow themselves to act almost without thinking, freeing up their conscious minds to note slight deviations or discrepancies from the norm, and to anticipate and head off problems well in advance. If you are still not convinced, think of yourself driving now, compared to when you first learnt. Most of what you do, you don't even realise you are doing.

This automation is fine, and indeed it is a vital part of becoming a skilled and integrated practitioner, but it is not fine if we inadvertently automate ineffective behaviours. If our perspective and values are set and clear in our minds then our

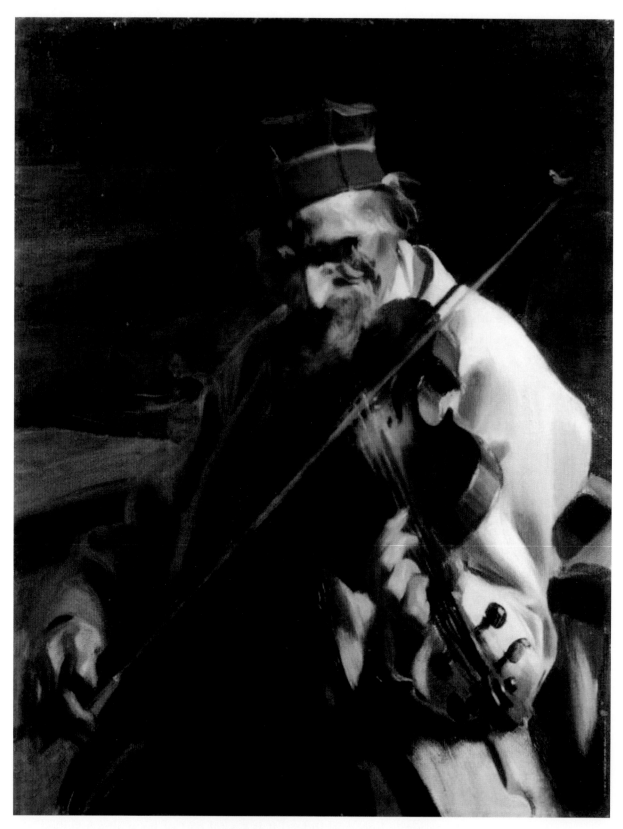

'Hins Anders' – by Anders Zorn (1904). Acting skilfully involves automating effective behaviours and not ineffective ones.

thoughts, words and actions have a much better chance of 'flowing'[22] efficiently and effectively. It is only when we have not integrated that we become slow and ineffective – as we are always finding internal dissonance and external opposition to our practice.

It is therefore not just desirable but crucial that we occasionally spend some time and effort reflecting methodically on what we do. That will help us to identify actions that are not 'righteous' – that is, actions that are neither 'right' nor 'wise' – in helping us to achieve those goals to which we have dedicated and committed ourselves.

BEING GOOD ENOUGH

That is not to say we can reasonably aim for perfection. A brilliant violinist may be so attuned to her music as to be able to let her fingers move without thinking, but she is aware enough to be able to identify mistakes she makes, wise enough to recognise that she can improve, and humble enough to realise she will never achieve perfection. It is the balance and interplay between that automation, awareness, wisdom and humility that makes her so brilliant.

Many health professionals tend towards perfectionism.[23] While setting high standards and being thorough are important elements in being an effective practitioner, perfectionism creates big problems.[24]

Perfection is an unattainable goal, so dedicating oneself to it is to dedicate oneself to failure. In that sense, perfectionism can be seen as a form of self-harm.

> Aiming for failure (by dressing it up as seeking perfection) is understandable.
> We are often more frightened of our potential than we are of our weakness.

Aiming for failure is not skilful as it reduces our self-esteem, shuts us into a continuous loop of dissatisfaction, makes us more likely to burn out, and closes us off to the possibility of mistake making. If we don't accept and embrace our mistakes, we cannot grow and develop.

Activity 5.2: The perfectionist game (30 minutes)

In order to see how perfectionist you are, try this test, called 'The Top Ten Signs Your a Perfectionist' (Flett 2004).
1. You cannot stop thinking about a mistake you made.
2. You are intensely competitive and can't stand doing worse than others.
3. You either want to do something 'just right' or not at all.
4. You demand perfection from other people.
5. You will not ask for help if asking can be perceived as a flaw or weakness.
6. You will persist at a task long after other people have quit.
7. You are a fault-finder who must correct other people when they are wrong.
8. You are highly aware of other people's demands and expectations.
9. You are very self-conscious about making mistakes in front of other people.
10. You noticed the error in the title of this list.

If you think you may have tendencies towards perfectionism (and if you are a practitioner there is a good chance you will), reflect for a few minutes on the strengths and weaknesses of your perfectionism. In what ways does it make you a better and happier practitioner; and in what ways does it make you a worse and less happy one?

It is not easy to drop perfectionism, as it is often a deeply ingrained belief and value, made deeper by a lifetime of habit-forming practice. We automate it, and self-harm is not a skilful thing to automate.

So maybe we need to start small, perhaps deliberately doing unimportant tasks imperfectly; such as using poor grammar or spelling. Try acting out in your imagination what an imperfect you would be like, and what kind of life it would be for you. When dissonance emerges, try not to get sucked into it, but observe and follow it, trying to find its source. Instead of telling yourself off for things that are not done perfectly, congratulate yourself for things done well.

When we can achieve the perspective that 'good enough is good enough' we create realistic, relational boundaries that are tough enough for our personal protection, but leaky enough to allow us to be compassionate and open as patient needs and work circumstances change.

Being 'good enough' can be difficult. It means deflating our egos and accepting that, whatever we do, we will never make more than a tiny difference in the face of the magnitude of the suffering that is in the world. But as our egos deflate, we find that we can take a healthier perspective. We can be content with the small difference we can make for the small number of patients we do care for. We can allow ourselves to be happy that we are only one of many, and that many can achieve much.

We may fool ourselves that perfectionism is a noble thing, but in reality it is the opposite. It is the fearful marriage of arrogance to self-harm. It is the setting-up of the self for failure, under the pretence that the self is able to achieve the unachieveable.

Being good enough is much harder, as it involves the truthful self-appraisal of our own strengths and weaknesses, and the courage to step into the world depsite those weaknesses, daring to trust in our own potential whatever troubles and obstacles lie ahead. In short, to live.

To be, or not to be, that is the question:

Whether 'tis nobler in the mind to suffer

The slings and arrows of outrageous fortune,

Or to take arms against a sea of troubles,

And by opposing end them? To die, to sleep,

No more; and by a sleep to say we end

The heart-ache, and the thousand natural shocks

That flesh is heir to: 'tis a consummation

Devoutly to be wished. To die, to sleep;

To sleep, perchance to dream — ay, there's the rub:

For in that sleep of death what dreams may come,

When we have shuffled off this mortal coil,

Must give us pause — there's the respect

That makes calamity of so long life.

For who would bear the whips and scorns of time,

The oppressor's wrong, the proud man's contumely,

The pangs of disprized love, the law's delay,

The insolence of office, and the spurns

That patient merit of the unworthy takes,

When he himself might his quietus make

With a bare bodkin? Who would fardels bear,

To grunt and sweat under a weary life,

But that the dread of something after death,

The undiscovered country from whose bourn

No traveller returns, puzzles the will,

And makes us rather bear those ills we have

Than fly to others that we know not of?

Thus conscience does make cowards of us all,

And thus the native hue of resolution

Is sicklied o'er with the pale cast of thought,

And enterprises of great pith and moment,

With this regard their currents turn awry,

And lose the name of action.

— *Hamlet* (Shakespeare)

Hamlet's soliloquy 'To be or not to be' occurs in the context of his considering suicide. Each time I read the text, I get something different, and to be honest I don't really understand it. But it came to me when writing this chapter, perhaps because I see perfectionism as a form of suicide. By removing all possibility of success, it kills life. The alternative, to 'grunt and sweat under a weary life' in a messy, imperfect and sometimes chaotic universe is not easy, so it is no wonder that our 'native hue of resolution' is occasionally 'sicklied o'er'. But it is in the messy, complex and sometime painful universe that we and our patients live, and so it is there we must practise, if that is truly what we wish for.

To be, or not to be, indeed.

THE 80:20 RULE

The 80:20 rule (also called the Pareto principle)[25] suggests that 80% of the effects of any action come from the first 20% of effort made. In other words, actions offer diminishing returns of effectiveness in a spiral of infinite regress, such that perfection can never be attained.

We may not be convinced that compassion for ourselves is sufficient reason to drop perfectionism. Therefore the Pareto principle may be more helpful in that it provides a rational reason for us to stop being perfectionists. The reason is that perfectionism is neither skilful nor effective.

If we try to achieve one task to 100% perfection, we will never reach it; we will exhaust ourselves, and so become less effective practitioners. If, however, we spread ourselves a little less deeply we will be able to spread ourselves much more widely, and achieve more results, more effectively for more patients.

I discovered this rule around the age of 17, and used it to justify to my horrified mother why I would only need to put 20% of my total effort into each of my three school exams, on the basis that 80% would be a good pass mark, and just enough to get me to university. I also calculated, but didn't mention, that it would still leave 40% for me to use for leisure and pleasure (girls, football and music, in no particular order) – which were far more enticing and enjoyable. In the event, I just scraped over the bar, scoring two Bs and a C, and taking advantage of the fact that medical schools were setting grades very low at that time (you need 3 As now). I was lucky to get away with my complacency as it turns out my logic was wrong and the maths doesn't actually work like that (which I may have worked out if I'd put a bit more effort into my maths...).

INTEGRATING AND BALANCING A RIGHTEOUS LIFE

There are many ways to be righteous, but they usually entail integrating our perspectives, beliefs and values with our choices, actions and words. As health practitioners we are very fortunate to work in a career where we can practise compassion and get paid for it. However, as health practitioners we are dealing with human health, so we cannot afford to be either complacent or arrogant.

In real-life health practice, however, there is at least one copper-bottomed guarantee. We will fail from time to time (*and in my case significantly more often than that*). But, to use the words of Ketut,[26] as long as we keep our head in the heavens, our feet on the ground, and a smile in our hearts, we won't go too far wrong.

Activity 5.3: Integration and balance (30 minutes)

Find a peaceful place and some quiet time, allow your worries and tensions to flow out, and meditate for a while on the picture.[27] Notice that the character has four feet, firmly planted on the ground, his head lost in heaven, and a gentle smile in his heart. Reflect for a while on your feet, your head, and your heart. Where are they?

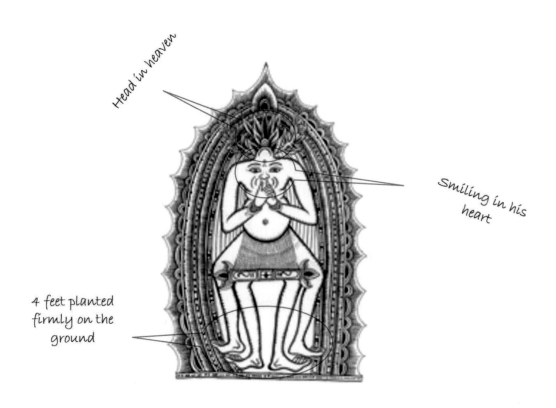

Head in heaven

Smiling in his heart

4 feet planted firmly on the ground

Chapter 6
Becoming aware and mindful

If you chase two rabbits, you catch none.

– Confucius

Activity 6.1: A bad day (30 minutes)

Cast your mind back to the last 'bad day' you had at work. Let your mind re-enact it and try as much as possible to 'be there'. Start to look inside and become aware of what was going on in your head at the time. Chances are it was noisy. Worries, frustrations, pressures, tiredness, emotions: all crowding and crowing for your attention. Try to remember them.

Now let your mind move outwards, towards the patients, colleagues or tasks you were dealing with at the time. How did you do? Not good? No doubt you were distracted, and as a consequence things were more clunky, irritating and inefficient than usual.

Does all that sound familiar? It certainly does to me, and I suspect to almost all of us.

The main elements of our practice are what we say and what we do. However, before either of these actions occurs, we actually carry out two more steps, so automatically and so quickly that we may not even notice them.

1. Becoming aware: of what is going on, both within and without.
2. Becoming mindful: clearing our minds before focusing on the matter in hand.

As practitioners, it is these two steps that we often seem to skip over. Yet, for all our emphasis on speed, efficiency and effectiveness in modern healthcare, it is these two steps which probably make all the difference between focused, efficient, effective practice and unfocussed, inefficient and ineffective practice.

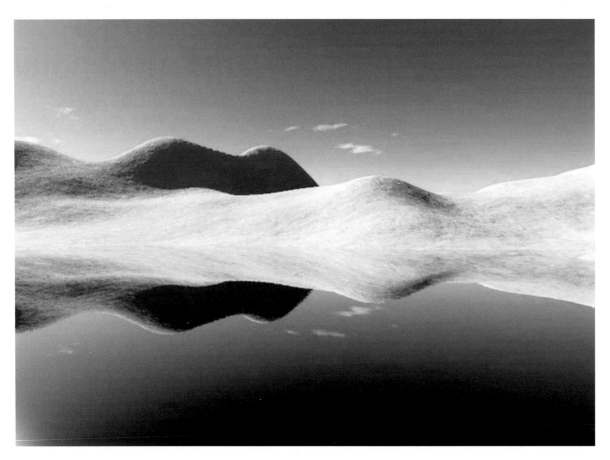

Clarity

AWARENESS

Being aware, being 'in' this moment means being 'not in' other moments (past or future), nor 'in' other thoughts and worries, nor 'in' other imaginary places or situations. It means stilling our minds and, in a calm and poised way, watching closely and listening deeply – not just to what is going on 'out there', but also to what is going on 'in here'.

True awareness is effortless. It takes no effort to watch the clouds drift by, to listen quietly to a bird singing, or to enjoy the smell of baking bread.

Awareness is 'shutting down' so that we can open up. We are not thinking, guessing, worrying or analysing. We are simply watching and listening to what is going on within and around us, and watching and listening to ourselves watching and listening.

In the sensory realm, we cannot stop our sensory apparatus sending data to our brains, unless we inhibit them with drugs or surgery. However, we can and do, albeit subconsciously, put all sorts of barriers in the way of fully open awareness; for example, ruminations, agitations and distractions.

Because we are not fully aware, we may miss or misinterpret the information we receive.

Without awareness we cannot properly assess our patients. If we are distracted the resulting misinterpretations can set us off into many a wild goose chase, which can leave the patient with his or her needs unmet; with our surgeries backlogged (as we waste time trying to recover lost ground); with our colleagues frustrated at our delay; our insurers charging us even higher premiums; and with us becoming frustrated and angry at ourselves and at our patients.

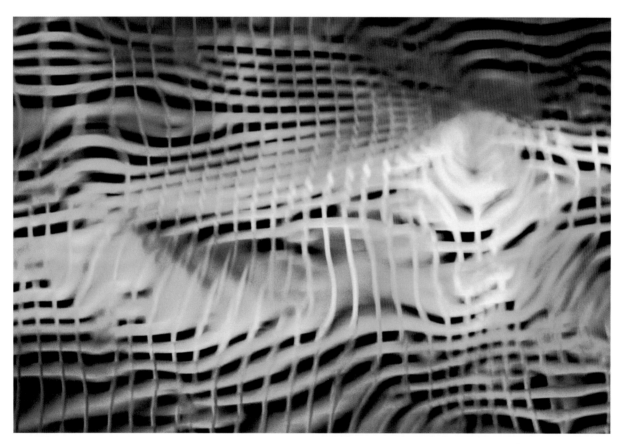

Distortion[28]

MINDFULNESS

We have all had the experience of seeing something familiar but as if for the first time: for example, a sunset, a starry sky, or the face of one we love. At such moments we truly 'see' something, giving it all of our single-pointed, focused attention. This is called mindfulness.[29]

At times like this, decluttering one's mind is one of the easiest and most pleasant things one can possibly do. It is as simple as quietly listening to one's breath, watching the clouds float across the sky, or absorbing beautiful music.

If you let cloudy water settle, it will become clear. If you let your upset mind settle, your course will also become clear.[30]

Nature that is around us, and consciousness that is within us, constantly generate amazing and wonderful things, thoughts and ideas. We often fail to notice them, because our attention is distracted and multi-focused rather than single-pointed.

Sometimes we like to talk about multitasking. There is no doubt that multitasking is extremely useful in the organised chaos of what healthcare can become. But there is a big difference between multitasking and being distracted.

Jugglers can juggle many balls, but they focus on one ball at a time, with their whole, mindful focus, one moment after another. They practise and practise until the whole thing becomes so automated, they could not even describe what they are doing or how they are doing it.

When walking, walk. When eating, eat. When listening, listen.

It sounds hard, but we all do it all the time. Actions like walking, or talking, take many months of hard labour (and bruises) for us to learn when we are babies. As adults, we do them without even being aware of them. Our thoughts and actions have become 'habits'.

BECOMING MINDFULLY AWARE

All thoughts and emotions are things, and mindfulness focuses on the no-thing. It looks for the gap between the images, the silence between the sounds. Once we become aware of that clear emptiness, we can allow it to absorb into our bodies and sink into our hearts, so bringing clarity to our minds.

In the bedlam of health practice, that clarity is a priceless resource. We can use our clarity to become aware of all the sense data we are receiving; to put all our observations into their rightful perspective, and to choose our words and actions wisely.

FLOWING

Flow[31] is the name for the state we sometimes feel when we are completely absorbed and immersed in what we are currently doing. In that state time and space seem to stand still, and we seem to move in slow motion, but in an incredibly efficient and effective way. It is possibly the ultimate state to be in for successful achievement, as all our focus and effort is single-pointedly targeted on the task in hand.

It is therefore an ideal state for us to try to achieve in practice.

Certain things, like apathy, agitation, boredom, depression and anxiety, will block flow states. On the other hand, we are more likely to enter a flow state if we are involved in an activity we enjoy, where there are clear goals, where we are engaged in a task requiring high challenge and high skill (but where there is a good balance between the size of the challenge and the level of our skill to meet the challenge – *see* the graph in the image below), and where we can get rapid and ongoing feedback so we can adjust as we go.

We cannot force ourselves into flow states, but we can significantly enhance our chances of achieving them by practising mindful awareness, single-pointed focus and active relaxation as we work. The effects of being in a flow state in health practice are hugely positive. We will be far more efficient and effective in what we do; we will notice more; we will make sharper and more conscious decisions; and the flow state will give us a deeper sense of joy and fulfilment.

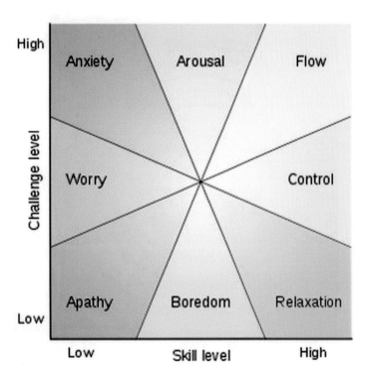

This graph[32] shows the relationship between challenge and skills. Low-challenge/low-skill tasks make us apathetic or bored. Medium-challenge tasks can make as anxious and agitated if we don't feel up to them. If we do feel up to them we feel relaxed and in control. As the challenge increases we become more aroused and eventually enter the flow state.

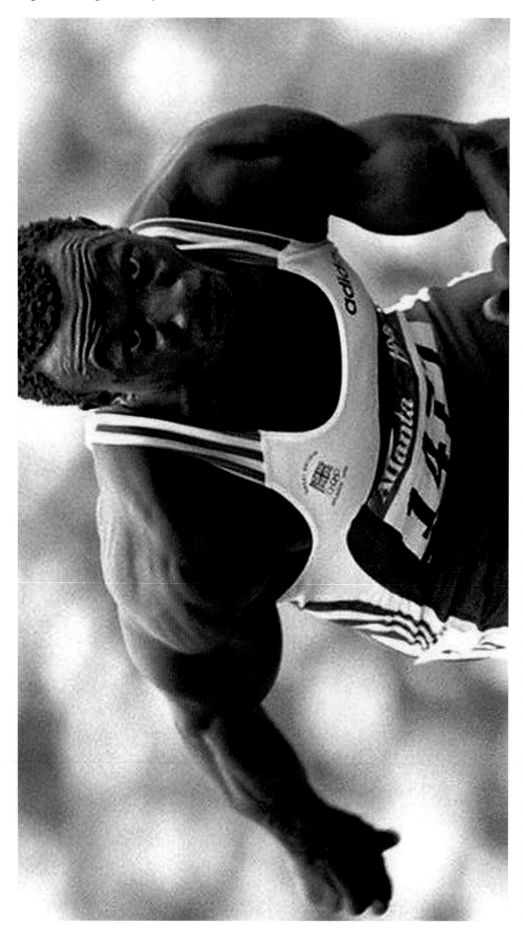

Linford Christie in the Olympic 100 metres final – absolutely absorbed and focused entirely on the winning line. (He won). Finding and maintaining a flow state in health practice is not a nebulous or airy-fairy concept. It makes for highly effective and efficient practice.[33]

WHEN OUR MINDS WON'T SETTLE

Sometimes, no matter how hard we try, we cannot get our minds to clear. It takes practice to stop our thoughts crowding in. On some days, our minds can seem 'as noisy as a barrel full of monkeys'. The trick is to observe them from a distance but not be drawn into them, allowing them to pass across our consciousness like clouds in the sky or fish slipping past in the depths of a still pool.

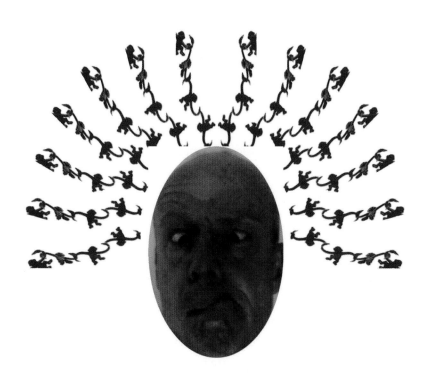

Activity 6.2: Awareness exercise (30 minutes)

Assume an erect and dignified posture. Then ask yourself: 'What is going on with me at the moment?' Simply allow yourself to observe whatever happens. Label any thoughts that you have and then leave them alone. Don't engage with them but just let them float away. Attend to your breathing or simply take in your surroundings instead.

Besides thoughts, there may be sounds that you hear, or bodily sensations that you are aware of. If you find yourself constantly elaborating on thoughts, rather than labelling them and returning to neutral, remember to observe your breathing. When emotions or memories of painful events occur, don't allow yourself to become caught up by them. Give them short labels such as 'that's a sad feeling', 'that's an angry feeling' and then just allow them to drift or float away. If you are patient, avoid getting cross with yourself, and smile gently at any failures you make, these memories and feelings will gradually decrease in intensity and frequency.

ILLNESS

As health practitioners, we are not immune from illness, and in fact we are more likely to suffer 'mental' illness than almost any other profession.[34] When suffering with anxiety, depression, substance abuse, eating disorders, obsessional-compulsive disorder, psychosis or any other form of mental illness; it is very hard to achieve mindfulness or to pull ourselves back from the edge.

At these times, we need to be honest and compassionate with ourselves. If we force ourselves on, we are at risk of harming ourselves, our patients and our organisations. Instead, we might hope to be as professional and systematic in identifying and addressing the problems with ourselves as we would be with patients.

It is better to seek objective and independent help, from our own health practitioners. If this is difficult, it can be worth looking at some of the available illness inventories to get a more objective feel for our state of mind. There are a number of these, for anxiety, depression, phobia, substance abuse, and a link is included in the endnotes.[35]

> I am talking from personal experience here, having become unwell several years ago. One of the earliest signs was an inability to get my mind to settle. Thoughts moved from being irritating to intrusive and then almost tyrannical, refusing to leave even when I wanted to settle. I lost all perspective, and felt lost to a maelstrom of negative thoughts, emotions and sensations. I therefore know from personal experience that it is very difficult to pull back once our minds become like this. It is tempting to just carry on and hope for the best. But these options are manifestations of God or Martyr complexes (which we will look at in more detail next chapter), and it is neither wise nor skilful to ignore them and hope they will go away.

Obsessions

Don't stop, can't stop, won't stop,
Think, think, think.
Running fast, running hard,
Don't know where.

Destination?
What a joke.
Just the road,
Just the speed

– JA

When feeling like this, it can be helpful to remind ourselves of the overall perspective of everything. Even if we worked every hour of every day, we would hardly scratch the surface of human suffering. We owe it to our patients, our colleagues, our families and ourselves to get healthy and stay healthy.

To recover we need to rest, to allow ourselves to show weakness, to ask for support[36] and to allow someone else to help us to find health again. Work will carry on without us, and, if it falls to pieces, it was not a healthy service to start with.

When we are unwell, it is easy to slip into thinking we are alone. But it is crucially important to realise we are not alone. We may be single, have few friends, or without close family. But we are not alone. We are surrounded by people, many of whom, like us, want to care for us and know how to care for us. Many others are in that position now, and many have been. They have recovered and we can.

It is very hard to admit to ourselves something is wrong. It is still harder to lay ourselves at someone else's feet, and ask for help. Looking back now, from a safe distance, I can see that I was getting increasingly unwell in the months leading up to my 'breakdown'. I had been writing more poems than usual, and they were dark and cynical. However, even though I was doing the writing, and even though I was doing the reading, I still did not have the awareness to realise what was happening to me.

Once it started, I was pretty much a wreck for several weeks, too frightened and tearful even to leave the house. I had little choice except to ask for help. But, as I did, I found that many, many people offered love, care and support. That was truly amazing to me, as I had always found my own weakness repulsive. However, that, more than anything else, was what helped me to recover. It made me realise that my fall into my abyss, terrifying as it was, was simply an opportunity to learn that I would be caught and held by the love and care of others.

This was a profound, albeit extremely welcome, shock to me. I had finally come to understand the only person standing in the way of my health and happiness was my own ego.

There was nothing for it: I had to go.

Letting go, and allowing others to catch me, was an act of egoistic self-destruction. My ego was very powerful, and so it is not surprising it didn't want to let go. But that egoistic destruction turned out also to become an act of self-creation. Falling off my own pedestal was painful but also liberating, because it freed me from the need to pretend to be any better than I was, and allowed me to accept that other people's love and care can truly be unconditional. Which is a bit mind-blowing, when you really think about it.

Tender

New Year's Day and new life start
Blinding light off frosted bark
Saplings reach to piercing blue
Tiny wren sings fearful tune
Gunshot ice crack splinters calm
Tender plant unsafe from harm

Age-old armour falls away
Weak and naked as my first day
Cast off skin lies at my feet
Tender senses reach to meet
The pains and joys that flood in
To opened heart as life begins.

Eased by love's healing balm
The warm embrace of gentle arms
Friends' soothing presence calms my mind
A world-proof fortress warm and kind
Angels guard me as I lay
Tender, safe on New Year's Day

– JA

Activity 6.3: Depression self-test (30 minutes)

Even if you are feeling fine, have a go at one of the depression or anxiety self-tests. This one is from the 'Black Dog Institute'. Please have a look at the website (www.blackdoginstitute.org.au) for a lot more useful information and resources.

	Not	Slightly	Moderately	Very
Are you stewing over things?				
Do you feel more vulnerable than usual?				
Are you being self-critical and hard on yourself?				
Are you feeling guilty about things in your life?				
Do you find that nothing seems to be able to cheer you up?				
Do you feel as if you have lost your core and essence?				
Are you feeling depressed?				
Do you feel less worthwhile?				
Do you feel hopeless or helpless?				
Do you feel more distant from other people?				

Scoring: items are scored as follows: 0 – for 'Not True', 1 – for 'Slightly True', 2 – for 'Moderately True', 3 – for 'Very True'

Results: 9 or more – if you have been feeling this way for more than a couple of weeks, or if these feelings persist for more than a couple of weeks, and as a consequence your day-to-day functioning is impaired, there is a good chance that you are clinically depressed. There might be wisdom in you speaking to a general practitioner (primary care physician), trained mental health professional or whomever you seek medical advice from to clarify this possibility. **Less than 9** – your responses to these questions suggest that you are unlikely to be clinically depressed. If your situation does not improve you might consider answering this screening measure again.

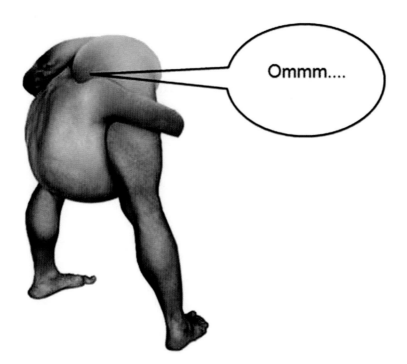

Ommm . . . When I first read about this stuff, I felt it was a load of baloney. I had enough to do without losing my head up my own a***. But, as time has gone on, I have become more and more aware of the cold, hard benefits of mindfulness in practice: more efficiency, effectiveness and job satisfaction.

PRACTISING MINDFUL AWARENESS

The practice of mindful awareness, as the name suggests, takes practice. It may be easy to do when we are relaxed, but it is much less easy to do when we are in a busy, hectic work environment; when we are unwell; when we are dealing with frightening emergencies; or when we are dealing with strong emotions.

There are many ways to practise mindfulness, and some of these are offered in the endnotes.[37] The common theme in all of them is learning how to physically and then mentally relax, begin to 'see' what is going on inside our minds, and then begin to dissociate from that activity, so we become witnesses as well as participants in our own activity, and aware of the full range of experiences in the present moment.

Rather like developing a second head.

If I were to pick out the one chapter in this whole series of books that would make the most difference to health practice, I think it would be this one. It is difficult to overestimate the value to health practice of being able to clear our minds very quickly (from moment to moment and patient to patient), to become mindfully aware of exactly what is happening within us and around us, and to move into a flow state within which the patient or task in hand has our full, single-pointed attention. As for me, I am still a novice. I can only manage to maintain this state for a small fraction of the time; but even that small bit has made a significant difference to my practice, my effectiveness, my efficiency and my enjoyment of my job.

To become mindfully aware takes practice. When we are practising awareness or mindfulness, we will definitely fall over. Hopefully, when we do, we can laugh at how silly we look when we fall off the wobbling bike, and smile kindly at ourselves when we have (yet another) go at climbing back on.

Ego

At first, when I fell off my pedestal

I thought I was seriously hurt

But in fact

All

I

Broke

Was my ego

– JA

Activity 6.4: Walking meditation (1 hour)

As health practitioners we hope to achieve a flow state when we are actually practising.

However, that is by no means easy, as real-life health practice is often chaotic, busy, noisy and full of distractions. *Well, mine is anyway.* So we will look at achieving flow states in actual practice later in this series. For now, it might be useful to start with something simple, which we can do without thinking and with few distractions – like walking.

To get the feel for a flow state in practice, try this 'walking meditation'. It is easy to remember, but you can read and record into your phone so you can listen to it as you go if you prefer.

Try to find a path that takes you through pleasing and relaxing scenery. Look up at the sky and breathe in, then, as you breathe out, let your distractions and tensions flow rapidly down through your feet into the ground. Take up a steady, but relaxing, pace. Allow yourself initially to become aware of any thoughts or emotions that might be tugging at your sleeve, wanting attention. Gently pat them on the head, and wave them off to play for a while. If they come back, smile and wave again.

As you step, be aware of the jog of your motion, and allow yourself to relax into a steady, pleasing rhythm. With each step, feel the earth initially resist, and then subtly mould to your step. Feel the gentle push it gives your foot as it leaves the ground.

Become aware firstly of the temperature. Whether it is warm, cold or hot, allow it to register on your skin, and absorb it. Enjoy that sensation for a while.

Start to gradually become aware of the fragrances around you. Let them wash around inside your temporal lobes for a while, evoking memories and taking you back, but not for long. Smile and wave off those memories, and simply enjoy the sensation of the fragrances, feeling them permeate into you.

Now become aware of the sounds. There are some loud sounds, hard to miss. Enjoy the shock of them, the way they resonate inside your head after they depart. Then start to listen for the silences between those sounds, and become aware of quieter sounds emerging. Enjoy the thrill of realising they too have been there all along, but are now making themselves available to you. Wave them off too, and listen to the silences between even the quietest sounds. Become slowly aware of an almost silent thrum, a deep, almost imperceptible energy, and then listen behind that too, to realise the deep silence behind all sounds. Immerse yourself in that deep silence.

Slowly allow the sounds to return, but smile and wave to them, because now you are becoming aware of the light. Initially, you can see things: people, plants, buildings, objects. As you walk, start becoming aware that there are many other, smaller things all around you. The details of a leaf; dust swirling in the breeze; the way the clouds are constantly but imperceptibly changing as they move; the gentle sway of a branch; the fleeting movement of a bird. Zoom out further, and instead of looking at things, start looking at the light. Notice the way it subtly changes as you move, colours shifting, and occasionally flashes through gaps, disappearing back into darker areas.

Then start looking deeper still, no longer looking at the light or at the things, but looking directly at the space between you and those things, at the emptiness through which the light moves.

Start to realise that this space is not absent but present. With every step you are emerging into it, moulding it, shaping it and then leaving it, to allow it to reform itself behind you. Enjoy the touch of nothing, as it moulds itself around you, and realise that as you walk along, you are forming and creating it as it is forming and creating you. It is a subtle, continuous dance. Immerse yourself in that dance for a while.

Slowly zoom back out, sensing everything, and sensing nothing. Drop deeply into the rhythm of your movement. Notice each breath, the rise and fall of your chest with the inflow and outflow of air, the warmth just inside your nose as you breathe out, and the coolness as you breathe back in.

As you walk feel more and more that you are making no effort, that you are being powered by nature itself. As though there is a force that is feeding every leaf, every building, every person, every bird and that this same force is powering you in your walking. Begin to feel that you are not separate from your surroundings but rather you are part of the surroundings that are walking with you.

Feel your awareness, and notice how you are aware of it. Smile at the nonsense of it, and enjoy your presence, your existence.

Chapter 7
Communicating effectively

Activity 7.1: Describing yourself with nouns (30 minutes)

While we are each individual and complete, we are also composite and many. In this chapter we will look at the idea of 'many me's'.

Start by thinking of, and maybe writing down, all the nouns that you or others use to describe you (e.g. 'mother', 'nurse' etc.).

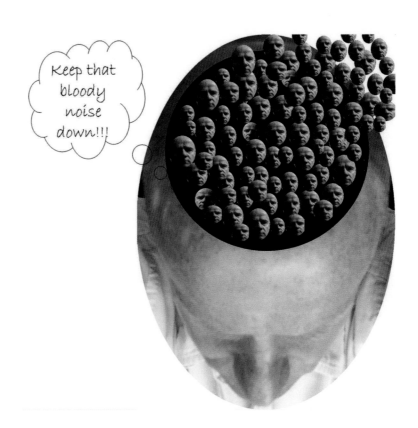

It may seem strange to have a chapter on 'communication' in the 'me' section. We normally think of communication as something that happens between people. However, from a relational perspective, we have many possible selves, each capable of generating perspectives, thoughts, emotions and ideas. Each of our selves is in constant communication with the others. So, for whatever reason, we seem to be able to have conversations with ourselves in a kind of 'society of the mind'.[38]

We are all aware of this phenomenon from the way we sometimes use reflexive language such as: 'I spoke before I could stop myself', or when we talk directly to ourselves 'for goodness sake, pull yourself together', or 'it seems ugly to me, but also beautiful in its own way'.

If you are interested in the theories of consciousness and language, please see workbook 5 (*Food for Thought*). For the purposes of the rest of this book, we will be focusing on practice rather than theory, so it doesn't matter too much what we believe, or the theory of how things work, ourselves included. The aim is to be practical and make the most of how we are, without worrying too much about the why.

Just as in the outside world, some of our internal voices can be very noisy and persistent, like a classroom full of children.

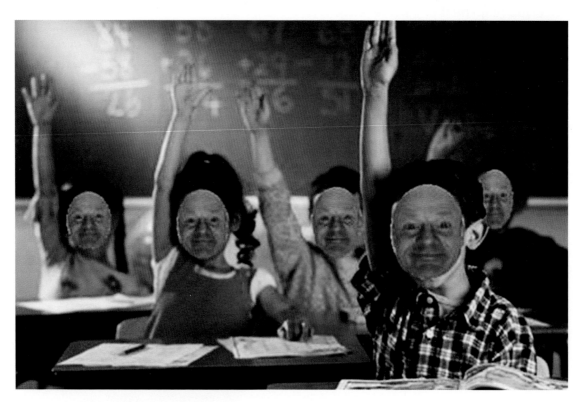

Once you begin to notice that you are more than 'one self', it tends to get a bit noisy inside your head. Trying to keep some discipline in among all the demanding voices is not always easy, but there are some benefits. Occasionally, some good ideas emerge. After all, many heads are better than one . . .

SELF-CONCEPTS

As health practitioners, we often have to hold, balance and integrate many different perspectives and positions within ourselves.

> For example: out of work I am a man, a dad, a husband, a son, a brother, and a friend. I am a frustrated 'greatest footballer the world has ever seen', a frustrated 'greatest tenor the world has ever heard', and seriously delusional. I am a shopper, a gardener, and a dog-walker. In work I am a doctor, an advocate, a gatekeeper, a judge, a counsellor, a teacher, a friend, and many more besides. In my subconscious I may be God, martyr, hopeless, good enough, narcissistic, anxious, self-confident, thoughtful, scatter-brained, a creation, a creator and a destroyer.

When we label and categorise ourselves like this, we create what is known as our self-concept.[39] Usually, we can hold a whole range of different self-concepts in tension, even when they are almost opposed to each other.

For example, when we were children, most of us hated bullying and being bullied. However, those of us with younger siblings will almost certainly have done a fair bit of bullying ourselves. That means they might have a self-concept that includes both 'being anti-bullying'; and also 'being a bully'. We may find it easier to think of ourselves as the first rather than the second. However, if we have a degree of insight, and are able to accept our own imperfections, we may be able to hold both of these apparently conflicting positions within our integrated self-concept.

As can be seen, reflective and projective narratives are relational. What I think will happen (my projective narrative) depends on who I think I am (my reflective narrative), but what then actually does happen either reinforces or contradicts who I think I am. The important point is that these dialogues and narratives are not just fictional creations of our minds, they are also the templates for our actual 'presents' and the foundations of our 'futures'.

Activity 7.2: Describing yourself with verbs (30 minutes)

While we might think of ourselves in nouns, 'who we are' may be better captured by what we do. After all, actions speak louder than words, and you can 'tell a tree by its fruit'. Think about some verbs that capture what you actually do in your day-to-day life, for example: 'healing', 'writing', achieving', 'worrying', 'rushing', 'comforting', 'ferrying' and so on.

Try writing down these verbs on a piece of paper and try to attach some of the nouns to these verbs. For example: I might link 'ferrying' to 'Dad'; or 'rushing' to both 'doctor' and 'dad'. Which verbs have lots of nouns attached, and which have few? What might these links tell you about yourself?

UNHEALTHY SELF-CONCEPTS

In some situations, some of our voices can dominate other voices, like classroom bullies. The dominated voices become quieter or become submerged altogether, so that we no longer hear them, even though they are still present and active subconsciously.

When we are not aware of, or become deaf to, the various voices of our 'mind societies', or if we are aware of them but do not balance them harmonically and in an integrated way, it can lead to 'splitting'[40] of our self-concept. Splitting is when we get subconscious conflicts between our various 'selves'. We often experience these conflicts as neuroses or as other unpleasant stresses or tensions.

Psychological splitting seems common in health professionals, so much so that particular types of split (or 'complexes') are recognised. These are as follows.

God complex

We can fall into the trap of believing that we are (or ought to be) supermen or superwomen, free of weakness. We can turn into obsessive, compulsive perfection-seekers; believing strongly in ourselves and our abilities; perceiving adverse events in the lives of our patients as personal failure; and divorcing ourselves from 'lesser mortals' such as patients and colleagues.

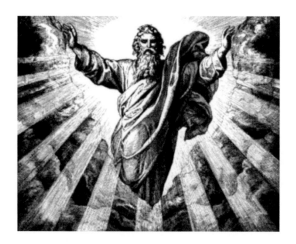

Martyr complex

We can also fall into the trap of identifying too strongly with the suffering of patients; feeling their pain and suffering as if it is our own; losing our personal boundaries and sense of perspective, and eventually becoming overwhelmed and exhausted by the pain.

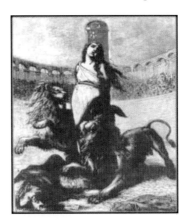

Messiah complex

This is a combination of both of the above, where we swing from one to the other moment by moment; alternately seeing ourselves as 'saviour Gods' saving our patients from illness, and then next as 'sacrificial martyrs' sacrificing our own health and happiness for our patients.

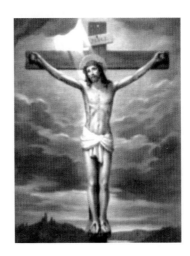

Repressed voices and positions such as these can start to 'act out' if we become overtired or overburdened. We may start by identifying too strongly with our patients, and perceiving unpleasant or adverse events in their lives as our personal failures. We may start to become tough with, or overcritical of, our colleagues, gradually losing the ability to see the world through anyone else's eyes, even our patients' eyes. As our compassion becomes exhausted we may start to express our 'shadow' sides, experiencing and expressing our work negatively, becoming ever more cynical and ever more distant from patients and colleagues.

Both of these complexes are traps that we might fall into through lack of awareness and lack of loving compassion for ourselves. As we have already seen, when we don't treat ourselves with loving compassion we may gradually 'burn out'. When we burn out we lose compassion for our patients, our colleagues, and our surroundings. We become ever more negative, hopeless, cynical, distant and resentful: threatening our job, our relationships, and our health and thereby removing from ourselves the very sources of happiness we need to survive and thrive.

INTERNAL NARRATIVES AND DRAMAS

Interestingly, the perspectives of narrative[41] and drama[42] can be quite enlightening in this context. These approaches explore the idea that, not only do we have internal dialogues (conscious or subconscious), but we also tell ourselves internal stories (or narratives) about ourselves and about the world around us; and we then act these narratives and voices out (as dramas), within and into our existence.

> *All the world's a stage,*
> *And all the men and women merely players;*
> *They have their exits and their entrances,*
> *And one man in his time plays many parts.*
>
> *– As You Like It* (Shakespeare)

We will deal with narrative and drama in more detail in workbook 2 (*Co-creating in Health Practice*). In summary, however, our internal narratives may be self-created from our own experience, or they may be passed on to us from our culture or our family or our religion. Our narratives help us to make sense of our experiences, and act as templates for future thoughts, choices and actions. Some of these narratives may be helpful and others not helpful.

Narratives may be 'reflective'. These are stories that we tell ourselves about how and who we are.

> For example: 'I am useless at biochemistry, always have been and I always will be' is a story that is not helpful before a biochemistry exam. Another story may be: 'Biochemistry is a logical process. I can be logical, so there is no reason I can't do biochemistry.'

Narratives can also be 'projective'. These are stories we tell ourselves about how things will be.

For example, an unhelpful story might be 'I have no chance of passing that biochemistry exam', whereas a more helpful story might be 'As long as I learn, practise, get some help when I am stuck and stay calm, I should be able to pass that biochemistry exam.'

Activity 7.3: Adding adjectives and adverbs (60 minutes)

Verbs and nouns give us the plot, but adverbs and adjectives bring narratives and dramas to life. Think about the words you commonly use to describe yourself and your actions (both publicly and privately). Begin to write them down under two headings: adjectives and adverbs. For example, under adjectives I might write 'effective' or 'hopeless' or 'useful'. Under adverbs I might write 'seriously', or 'irritatingly' or 'calmly'.

Now try and look at yourself from the perspective of other people: your family, your friends, your colleagues, strangers and so on. Start thinking about and noting down the adverbs and adjectives they might commonly use about you. Compare those to the words you have written about yourself.

Finally, start pulling together common public and private narratives about yourself from all of the words (nouns, verbs, adjectives and adverbs). For example, 'She is a caring nurse who practises compassionately'. 'I am a worrier who is always concerned about how others might judge me' or 'I am usually right'.

Reflect on these narratives. How easily do they weave together to create the 'composite you'? Are they mainly working together, or are they in conflict? How might this together-ness or conflict play out in your actual life and experience of living as a person and as a practitioner?

UNHEALTHY VOICES AND NARRATIVES

An example of one story that we health practitioners often tell ourselves (and then act out as a real-life drama) is that of the 'wounded healer'.[43] Many of us may have a history of past events or relationships that have hurt us in some way; for example, loss, bereavement, caring for unwell relatives, abusive or dysfunctional family or personal relationships.

Being skilful and compassionate with ourselves means acknowledging and accepting our own pain, loss and weakness. If we do not acknowledge and accept them, we may end up repressing them, and psychologically splitting. When we are psychologically split, our repressed 'shadow sides' may negatively (and subconsciously) influence our thoughts, our narratives or our actions (when stories get acted out as 'dramas').

One narrative and drama that got acted out to terrible effect was that of Harold Shipman, a much loved, intelligent, dedicated, apparently gentle, and well-respected family doctor in Lancashire. It is very sobering to consider and reflect upon what the voices, complexes and narratives must have been in order for him to justify to himself the killing of 200 of his patients.

I wake and feel the fell of dark, not day.
What hours, O what black hours we have spent
This night! what sights you, heart, saw; ways you went!
And more must, in yet longer light's delay.
With witness I speak this. But where I say
Hours I mean years, mean life. And my lament
Is cries countless, cries like dead letters sent
To dearest him that lives alas! away.

I am gall, I am heartburn. God's most deep decree
Bitter would have me taste: my taste was me;
Bones built in me, flesh filled, blood brimmed the curse.
Selfyeast of spirit a dull dough sours. I see
The lost are like this, and their scourge to be
As I am mine, their sweating selves; but worse

– Gerard Manley Hopkins

INTEGRATING VOICES, NARRATIVES AND DRAMAS

Health practice is not easy work, but it is rewarding work. Unbalanced narratives and dialogues lead to unbalanced and unsettled minds, and eventually to unbalanced and unskilful practice.

It may well be that we have experience of past pain, or that we have complexes, or that we are psychologically split, or that we tell ourselves unhelpful stories, or that we act out in ineffective ways. In fact, it is very unlikely that we do not have some or all of these. Pretending otherwise is unhelpful, and may even be dangerous, to our patients and to ourselves.

However, we don't have to view these complexes or narratives negatively. On the contrary, we can turn each of these to our advantage and use them to become more skilful practitioners. Experience of pain and damage, and awareness of their consequences, can make us far more compassionate, aware and effective practitioners.

The difference between skilful and unskilful health practice may be seen as the practice of compassionate self-awareness. When we become compassionately self-aware of our voices, narratives and dramas, we give ourselves the best opportunity to gain mastery of them, rather than the other way around. As we gain mastery of them we can begin to transcend them and use them as worthwhile platforms for personal development and improved practice.

Past experiences that are painful can be very helpful in our work because they can help us to be more empathic and better able to understand and communicate with people who are sick or dying. Compassionate awareness of our vain complexes can bring us some humility and free us from the terrible drain of constantly fighting and repressing our shadow sides. Personal experiences of acting out dramas unskilfully can become rehearsals for far more skilful performances in practice.

A USEFUL TOOL – JOHARI WINDOW

Johari window is a tool for improving mindful self-awareness. The window represents all possible information about 'me'.

1. My 'Open Area'	3. My 'Blind Spot'
2. My 'Hidden Area'	4. The 'Unknown'

5. Nothingness

The Johari window (adapted)

As we look through the different panes of this window, directing our gaze at ourselves, we will get five different perspectives (although the creators of the window only described four – they did not mention the background 'nothingness', so I have added that). The Johari window 'panes' can be changed in size to reflect the relevant proportions of each type of 'knowledge'.

1. If we look through the open window, we will see what we already know about ourselves, and which we have shown to others. This information is easily accessible, but we often need to remind ourselves to look.

How is my body these days? Which of my obvious needs am I neglecting? Am I getting enough sleep? When did I last have a really good laugh? In practice, do I ever audit or reflect on how I am doing?

2. If we look through the hidden area, we will see things we already know about ourselves, but which we have kept from others. We are already aware of this information, so we don't need any tools to become more aware of it. However, we may want to ask ourselves why we have hidden the information, as hiding is usually borne out of fear, and fear is rarely a helpful or skilful motivation in life (although there may be times when self-protection is crucial).

    What do I feel guilty about or ashamed of? Which situations make me happy, sad or mad? Which of my desires do I love but would not want to admit to others? What am I frightened of? What do I think will happen if I open up? In practice, what is it that makes me stressed? Do I ever catch myself playing God or martyr? What are the helpful and unhelpful ways I describe myself or the stories I tell myself?

3. If we look though the blind area, we will see nothing, because we are not conscious of it. However, we can open this area up by asking others for their (compassionate) description of what they see.

    What do my family and friends think about me? What are my characteristics and abilities? What do they most like about me and what do they find most off-putting? What situations do they think make me happy, or mad, or sad? What do my neuroses seem to be and how do my defences kick in? What do my patients think about me, or my colleagues? Can I ask them to give me some anonymous or open feedback? Can I use that feedback as a tool for self-development?

4. If we look though the unknown area, again we will see nothing, because we are not conscious of it. Unlike the blind area, other people cannot help here, as they are also blind to it.

    We cannot see what we are blind to, but we may be able to see the effects of our unconscious actions and behaviours. Reflecting critically and systematically on particular events can be helpful, either alone, or in supervision with a colleague. Practising non-attachment through meditation or contemplation, and watching what thoughts and emotions arise, can be helpful. Another way is to keep a diary of when we find ourselves reacting emotionally, and see if certain situations or themes keep cropping up. In practice, we could use the 'PUNS and DENS'[44] model, or significant events analysis.

5. If we look at the background to the window, and at the background to everything we see through the window, we will still see nothing, because there is nothing to see.

And in seeing the gaps and hearing the silences we realise that this is where our consciousness springs from, and to which it will return. Observing these gaps and listening to these silences will not tell us anything at all, as there is nothing there to be told. But it will allow clarity to develop, perspective to be attained, and peace to enter the room.

The practice of self-awareness and balanced integration involves changing the relative sizes of the different windows. As we become more open to the opinions and voices of others, window 2 begins to shrink. As we are less ashamed to act out who we are, warts and all, window 3 begins to shrink. As we become more aware of our 'shadow side', window 4 begins to shrink. As the others shrink, window 1 grows, and through window 1 the reality of our existence and practice can be clearly seen.

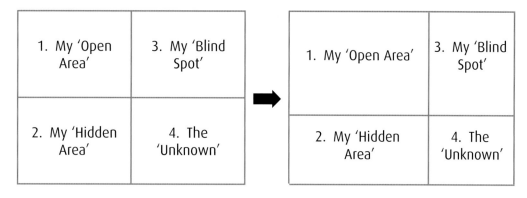

Building self-awareness and openness

5. Nothingness

COMMUNICATING WITH MYSELF SKILFULLY AND EFFECTIVELY

Once we become aware of the sheer range of voices, positions, dialogues and stories within us we can discover a huge potential for healthy self-creation. We can choose different voices or rewrite new stories whenever we want. We can add different characters, bring in different themes, or work out new endings. By using these as tools for healthier and more balanced self-creation, we open the opportunity for healthier and more balanced futures for ourselves in health practice.

This is not a woolly, airy-fairy approach. This is as important to our practice as being able to use drugs; or surgical techniques. We are the most important tools we have. An unbalanced or unstable tool is at best an ineffective tool, and at worst a dangerous one.

As we bring our voices and narratives into an integrated and harmonic whole, we reduce the noise and confusion in our minds, thereby allowing our minds to become clearer and ourselves to become more aware. When we are mindful and aware, we are in a better position to live healthy lives, and be healthy practitioners.

It is only with the heart that one can see rightly; what is essential is invisible to the eye.

— Antoine de Saint-Exupery

What lies behind us and what lies before us are tiny matters compared to what lies within us.

— Oliver Wendell Holmes

The kingdom of heaven is within you.

— Jesus Christ

He who knows himself, knows heaven.

— Mohammed

So doth heaven abide within thee, why search without?

— Vedas

Activity 7.4: 360-degree feedback with a difference (4 hours)

'Appraisal' has become rather a dreaded word (and narrative, and drama) for health practitioners, but it can be a tool as well as a tyrant. Most appraisals require us to get feedback from colleagues, and colleague feedback is probably the most accurate assessment of how we are doing. It can, however, be scary, and damaging if handled unskilfully or without compassion. It can also become a chore. However, we can be a bit creative and so keep it fresh and useful. Here are a few possibilities.

1. Ask a selection of 8–10 of your colleagues, friends and family only to provide verbs, or adjectives, or adverbs, or a combination (but no nouns) in your feedback and see how they compare to your own.

2. Ask a selection of 8–10 of your colleagues, friends and family to write brief narratives about you as they see you, and see how they compare to your own.

3. Complete your own Johari window, and then ask a selection of 8–10 of your colleagues, family and friends to do the same for you. Compare what is in each window. Which ones are 'really' you? What might be left in the 'blind spot?

Chapter 8
Acting skilfully

Activity 8.1: Remembering our needs (30 minutes)

Find a quiet place and moment, and gently but quickly scan down your body, loosening and relaxing any tight spots. Open the floor of your mind and allow your thoughts and emotions to flow away, enabling a few moments of clarity to emerge. In that space begin to become aware of yourself.

As you do, don't be concerned if you feel resistance, or emotion, or distraction. Defences are normal and healthy, but just now you don't need them. Allow them to flow away too, and look at yourself as you would at a new patient.

What is it that you need in order to survive and thrive? As each need emerges, note it then let it go. When no further ideas or images emerge, bring yourself gently back to the moment and note down your needs before you forget them.

ACTING WITH COMPASSION

Acting skilfully towards ourselves in practice means more than just acting with technical competence. It means applying our skills with love and compassion.

We don't mean this in a mushy way. Using one's love and compassion skilfully takes wise understanding of perspectives and values; clear and perceptive awareness of what is going on; strength to follow a righteous and just lifestyle; courage to be honest in what we say; and skilfulness in how we act.

We also may think that love and compassion is something we 'do' for other people. But before we can 'do' it for others, we have to 'do' it to ourselves.

For health practitioners like us, this may be very hard indeed, and involve undoing a lifetime of bad habits towards ourselves.

'Acting' skilfully in regard to ourselves means creating our present moment in a compassionate and effective way. If we create compassionate and effective present moments, we inevitably create compassionate and effective pasts and futures for ourselves.

ACTING SKILFULLY TOWARDS OURSELVES

If we adopt a compassionate and loving attitude to ourselves, we will create these positive moments naturally. If we can stay 'present' in the moment, they will naturally flow in a harmonious, balanced and integrated way.

In theory, therefore, there is no need to go over anything more in this chapter.

On the other hand, in the real world of health practice, the instances where we can really achieve that harmonious balance are few and far between. If and when we do stumble into the odd 'Zen' moment (where we feel completely at ease, connected and aware), it is over almost as soon as it has begun.

Therefore, it may be helpful to look at some of the ways we can act more effectively in relation to ourselves. This is not a selfish objective as we will not be able to help others become as balanced, integrated and harmonious as they can be unless we are as balanced, integrated and harmonious as we can be.

FULFILLING OUR NEEDS AND SETTING OUR GOALS

In thinking about how best to act towards ourselves, it may be helpful to have a structure from which to work. There are many we could use, and each gives useful insights, but perhaps the best known and most widely used is Maslow's 'hierarchy of needs'.[45]

Maslow suggests we each have needs, from very basic physiological needs, through to highly complex transcendence needs. Each higher need is founded upon the lower level needs, as described in the diagram below.

It might therefore be worth skimming through these needs, and reflecting on how well we meet them in our own lives.

Physiological needs

Our physiological needs are well known to us as health practitioners. However, we do not appear always to practise what we preach. These are the things our parents told us (*so it is very annoying to have to admit they were right*). It's a question of eating well, sleeping well, keeping fit, keeping supple, and going easy on caffeine, alcohol and other substances.

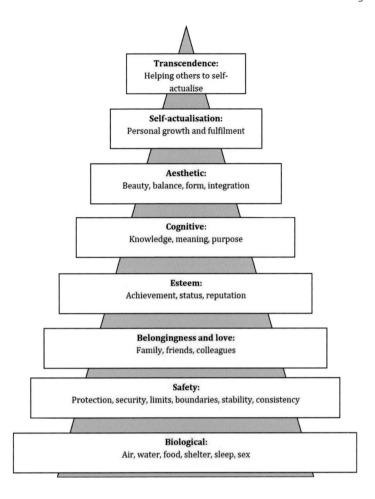

Maslow's hierarchy of needs – in diagrammatic form.

Safety needs

When we talk about safety, we often think about physical safety. Of course this is important. However, safety can be psychological as well as physical. We may feel threatened by financial worries, by abusive pasts or presents, by disorganisation or bullying at work, by chaotic work environments, or by insecure jobs. The more we try to protect ourselves, the more closed off we can become. But it feels very difficult to open up when we feel like we will be hit from all sides if we do. So it is important that we do our scenario-planning, and safety-netting; but if these become all-consuming, we will become blocked at this level, and not progress.

Activity 8.2: Safety needs (1 hour)

We may not think of health practice as being unsafe, at least not compared, say, to mining, or racing driving. but our morbidity (illness) and mortality (death) rates are high.

To give you an idea of how 'safe' your practice is, read through and reflect on the following questions. Better still, go to the Black Dog Institute website* and do it online, so you can compare yourself to others in your and other professions.

- Is your work fulfilling?
- In general terms, do you trust the senior people in your organisation?
- Do your daily work activities give you a sense of direction and meaning?
- At a difficult time, would your boss be willing to lend an ear?
- Does your work eat into your private life?
- Does your work bring a sense of satisfaction?
- Do you believe in the principles by which your employer operates?
- Is your boss caring?
- Do you feel stressed in organising your work time to meet demands?
- Does your work increase your sense of self-worth?
- Do you feel content with the way your employer treats its employees?
- Does your job allow you to recraft your job to suit your needs?
- Do you feel that your boss is empathic and understanding about your work concerns?
- Do you feel excessively pressured at work to meet targets?
- Does your work make you feel that, as a person, you are flourishing?
- Do you feel that your employer respects staff?
- Does your boss treat you as you would like to be treated?
- After work, do you find it hard to wind down?
- Do you feel capable and effective in your work on a day-to-day basis?
- How satisfied are you with your work's value system?
- Does your boss shoulder some of your worries about work?
- Do you find yourself thinking negatively about work outside work hours?
- Does your work offer challenges to advance your skills?
- Compared with your organisation's 'ideal values', to what degree are actual work values positive?
- Do you feel your transactions with your boss are, in general, positive?

- Do you feel that you can separate yourself easily from your work when you leave for the day?
- Do you feel you have some level of independence at work?
- Do people at your work believe in the worth of the organisation?
- Do you believe that your employer cares about their staff's well-being?
- Does your work impact negatively on your self-esteem?
- Do you feel personally connected to your organisation's values?

We will talk more about how to manage your workplace and colleagues later in the series but, for now, consider whether there is anything you can do to improve your sense of security at work. What do you have power to change? Do colleagues or bosses know how you are feeling? How can you wind down more effectively after work?

* www.blackdoginstitute.org.au/surveys/workwellbeing/index.cfm

Love and belonging needs

Small babies and children who are not loved find it very difficult to fully recover. Their brains wire up in such a way that they find it difficult to make loving and trusting relationships in later life. Love is therefore as important as food, drink and safety. We need to belong: to family, to peer groups, to cultures and societies, to professional teams. It is sometimes easy to take people we love (and groups we belong to) for granted, focusing too much on daily, but less important, distractions or commitments. Within our practice, we have an opportunity to belong, but also both to give and to receive love and compassion with our friends, our patients and our colleagues. In an environment where working relationships are not like that, it can be difficult.

But it is in giving that we receive.

Love

Love bade me welcome, yet my soul drew back,
Guilty of dust and sin.
But quick-ey'd Love, observing me grow slack
From my first entrance in,
Drew nearer to me, sweetly questioning
If I lack'd any thing.

'A guest,' I answer'd, 'worthy to be here';
Love said, 'You shall be he.'
'I, the unkind, ungrateful? ah my dear,
I cannot look on thee.'
Love took my hand, and smiling did reply,
'Who made the eyes but I?'

'Truth, Lord, but I have marr'd them; let my shame
Go where it doth deserve.'
'And know you not,' says Love, 'who bore the blame?'
'My dear, then I will serve.'
'You must sit down,' says Love, 'and taste my meat.'
So I did sit and eat.

– George Herbert.

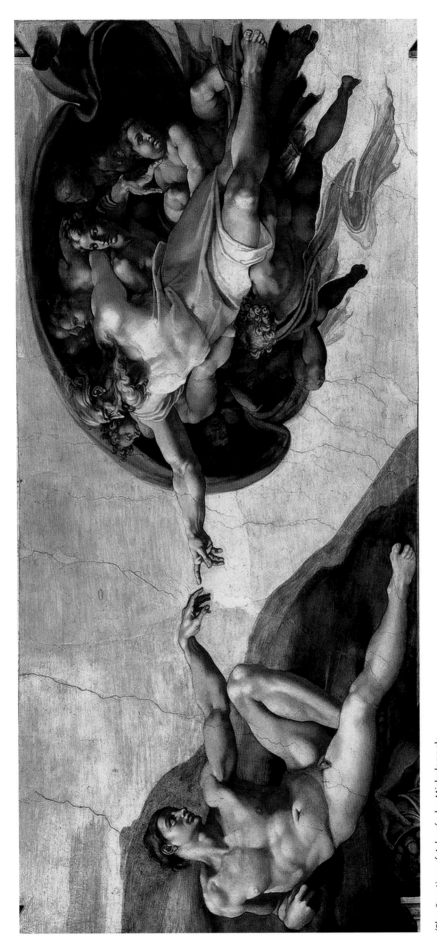

'The Creation of Adam' – by Michelangelo

Esteem needs

As health practitioners we are very fortunate in working in careers that other people look up to and respect. This gives us a strong sense of belonging, and a strong sense of personal value and acceptance. If we can avoid falling into God or Martyr complexes, we can take great and deserved pleasure from this respect, and allow ourselves to feel a sense of self-esteem. However, we will find it almost impossible to accept the esteem of others unless and until we can learn to accept and love ourselves 'internally'.

Again, we are very fortunate as health practitioners in that we have a wonderful opportunity to learn, develop and gain mastery of our practice. With increasing mastery comes increasing self-confidence and independence, and these give us ever greater opportunity to value ourselves as others value us.

Cognitive needs

We are born to learn. It is through learning that we develop our ability to express ourselves, to explore our worlds, to create meaning and to find understanding. As practitioners we have a tremendous opportunity for fulfilling this need to learn, not just through our initial training, but through ongoing exploration and development both within and through our practice.

Aesthetic needs

All work and no play make us dull boys (and girls). But aesthetics is not just about escape. It is about a different form of expression and creation. We create and admire visual and auditory images for many reasons, not least because they help us express and find meaning in ways that go beyond our ability to conceptualise, categorise and verbalise. Beauty both refreshes us and transports us, creating within us a sense both of connection and transcendence.

We do not always think of health practice in terms of beauty. Indeed as practitioners we have to witness and deal with some of the ugliest aspects of existence: death, violence, decay, corruption and loss. However, with a little thought, we can fairly easily find beauty in our work. The human body is a truly astonishing and beautiful creation; as is the sound of a newborn baby's cry, the touch of a grateful patient or the smile on the face of a child who has been freed from pain. The beauty is in front of us, as long as we can open our eyes to see it.

*A **thing of beauty** is a joy for ever*

A thing of beauty is a joy forever:

Its loveliness increases; it will never

Pass into nothingness; but still will keep

A bower quiet for us, and a sleep

Full of sweet dreams, and health, and quiet breathing.

Therefore, on every morrow, are we wreathing

A flowery band to bind us to the earth,

Spite of despondence, of the inhuman dearth

Of noble natures, of the gloomy days,

Of all the unhealthy and o'er-darkened ways

Made for our searching: yes, in spite of all,

Some shape of beauty moves away the pall

From our dark spirits.

– John Keats

Self-actualisation needs

In this workbook we have talked often about existence as a continuous process of self-creation. While many factors come together in relationship to form the 'Holon' we call 'me'; everything that we consciously experience is perceived, mediated and expressed through our consciousness, which is a self-created entity. So we literally create ourselves.

As we have a degree of control of our consciousnesses (in that we can make choices), we therefore have a degree of control about 'who' we choose to create ourselves to be. The 'who' we choose to be is created by a series of our choices and actions; some of which are conscious. As we have seen in earlier chapters, even automated and unconscious choices can be brought to our awareness and changed for the better. So, to an extent, we are who (and what) we choose to be.

In many ways this is a frightening concept. Of course we are constrained by our physical and biological structures and lifespan. We cannot go back and change the moulding experiences of our pasts. But we can create our futures. Even within the constraints of nature and nurture we have an infinite range of choices available to us. This ability to create ourselves confers upon us a tremendous responsibility, and that responsibility can be almost unbearable, so we often fall into denial: pretending that we are simply victims of the universe or of fate. We are of course victims of the universe, and maybe even of 'destiny' (whatever that is), but we are also masters of them too. Which is easier: to be a victim with no control, or a master with considerable control?

Health practice is demanding and difficult. Most of us are frightened of failing but, perhaps more subconsciously, we might be even more frightened of the potential we have to succeed. With perspective, value and mindful focus, if we communicate skilfully with ourselves, and take care of our fundamental needs, we have the potential to create and 'actualise' lives that are not just righteous but also healthy, happy and wise. This is a heavy responsibility, maybe even a curse, but it is also a tremendous opportunity and blessing too.

Transcendence needs

Maslow's initial model did not include transcendence, but he included it later in life.[46] When we realise that we are self-created, we may realise that we are also self-transcending. We have the ability to move beyond and out of the limitations of the 'self' and recognise our interdependence upon and inter-connection with the entire universe. In other words, we have the potential not just to 'actualise' ourselves, but we have the ability to actualise other entities and beings too, helping them reach ever higher levels and experiences of existence, and so of health. Again, this is a heavy responsibility but also a wonderful opportunity.

In health practice, perhaps more than any other profession, we have the unique privilege to witness and share in the creation, development, progress, decay and destruction of life. That gives us the opportunity, every now and again, to set aside the technicalities of what we do, and allow ourselves to address the many questions those experiences ask of our own existence, and of our own non-existence, seeking some enlightenment along the way.

The Wise Man

The wise man . . .
Sits alone in the desert, melting into the sands.
Floats alone in the ocean, dissolving into the depths
Lies alone in his coffin, easing into infinity.

– JA

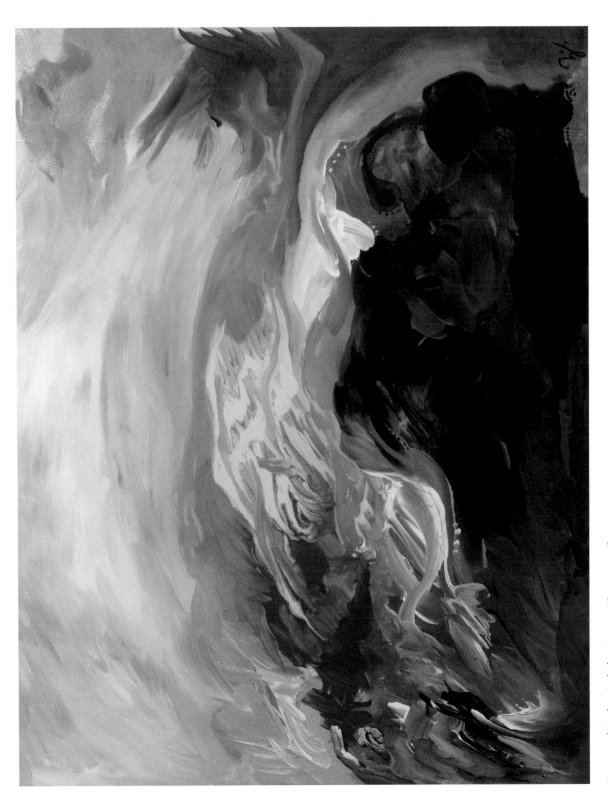

'Transcend Conformity' – by Sara Ann Zimmerman[47]

FINDING SATISFACTION IN OUR PRACTICE

When we act skilfully and compassionately with ourselves, we embark on a journey of self-discovery and self-expression. It is a journey that starts from infinite nothingness, and ends in infinite nothingness. We are of course restricted and constricted by the physical confines of our existence. But as sentient beings we still have an infinite number of choices about what we do between our births and our deaths, and about how we choose to do it.

So as practitioners we have a tremendous opportunity to find and fulfil all our needs, from basic through to transcendent. Health practice can therefore be not just a satisfying but an enriching and even enlightening career.

If we choose to treat ourselves with love and compassion, we give ourselves the best chance of creating an existence for ourselves that is integrated, harmonic and balanced. This life is ours, to create as we wish.

We must not cease from exploration. And the end of all our exploring will be to arrive where we began and to know the place for the first time.

– T.S. Eliot

Activity 8.3: Telling your story (1 hour)

Take some time to find a quite space, or maybe go for a walk. It doesn't matter, as long as you have time and space. Once your body is relaxed and your mind settled, start to tell your own story. If you like, actually start with 'Once upon a time'. Start with your earliest memories and gradually thread together a coherent narrative that brings you to today. Again, thoughts and emotions will arise. Smile and wave at them, and send them on their way. There will be many narratives, so don't worry if it is confusing. Just choose those you feel comfortable with.

Now look forward to your death, and complete your narrative. This time, come up with three different endings: a 'bad' ending, where your needs are hardly actualised at all, an 'OK' ending where some are, and a 'good' ending where they are nearly all actualised.

Then let the narratives evaporate into the ether. Come back to now. Consider your potential. Actually look at it, hear it and feel it. Don't be surprised if it is a bit frightening. Just get used to its presence for a while. Over the next few weeks, spend some minutes each day in its company and observe how it affects your views and choices.

Chapter 9

Health practice as self-practice

Activity 9.1: Self-creation (30 minutes)

As health practitioners, we tend to be cynical about so called 'New Age' ideas. Indeed you may think that 'self-creation' just another meaningless 'New Age' term. However, think again, but with your most rigorous, scientific and logical hat on.

Take a look at yourself. What do you see? A roughly human-shaped person, with a pinkish, olivey or brownish-coloured skin? Basically smooth but with hairy areas? Yes, but think again. If you looked at yourself in the dark, what colour would you be? If under a light microscope, would you be smooth? If under an electron microscope, would you have solid form? If in the Hadron Collider, how much of you would simply be space? If from space, would you exist at all?

The universe is relational, and it is made up of energy, forces and matter. Consider the apparent fact that our concept of self is entirely relational, and entirely contextual. Consider the logical conclusion that our idea and experience of personhood is a creation of our conscious minds.

Take a look inside. Can you find experiences of 'colour' or 'warmth' or 'beauty' or 'shape' or 'smoothness' or 'love'? Peep 'outside' again, looking at the universe with scientific eyes. Can you still see these experiences? Do they have physical correlates in the universe of matter, energy and forces?

Think on. Who are you? Imagine you had no consciousness of being alive. Other people could tie you down to a certain locus in space–time, and give you corresponding coordinates, but could you be said to 'exist' in the full, human sense of the word?

Consider the apparent fact that, while we are physical bundles of matter and energy in the space–time continuum, we have no other existence outside that which we are conscious of. What we are conscious of, our consciousness creates, within itself, in a closed, self-referential loop.

When we go about experiencing our existence (feeling warmth, and colour, and shape, and sounds, and vision, and beauty and love) these attributes and experiences are of our own creation. We create them as we go about existing, moment by moment.

In other words, in a very hard, concrete, scientific and real way, we create ourselves.

Here are two interesting observations about health practitioners:
- as conscious beings, we create ourselves
- as health practitioners, we are our own tools.

The combination of these two things is both a blessing and a curse.

It is a blessing because we are able to make choices that are skilful and wise, so that we are able to create a healthy, balanced and effective present; and so that we create a healthy, balanced and effective future. When we practise, we bring patients both into our presence and into our presents. If that presence and those presents are compassionate and skilful, both practitioner and patient can co-create a balanced and healthy shared present, from which both can come out of them more whole and more healthy.

It is a curse because it means we have a responsibility, not just to ourselves but to our patients. If we make unskilful choices, we create presence and presents that are unbalanced and unhealthy. When we bring patients who are in pain or damaged into our negative presence and into our negative presents, we co-create an unhealthy and unbalanced present, from which both come out less whole and less healthy.

There are many ways and means in which a practitioner may become more skilful at co-creating a shared consciousness, shared presents and individual futures in ways that heal rather than damage either the practitioner or the patient. These ways and means involve becoming aware of, managing and rebalancing oneself continuously: every morning, every patient, every experience and every year.

Being a professional health practitioner is therefore about more than just being technically competent. It is about being able to understand ourselves; knowing our strengths and points of weakness; being able to pace ourselves; and mastering how we use ourselves effectively, keeping ourselves sharp, enthusiastic and happy in our work.

Thus we have a happy confluence of duties. If we wish to discharge our duty to be effective practitioners, we have a duty to ensure we make ourselves happy in our work. Health practice is life-practice, and life-practice is health practice.

Caring for ourselves is therefore not an optional extra, or a sign of weakness, or of selfishness. It is a critical, perhaps **the** critical, skill that we have to master as health practitioners.

CREATING OUR OWN PRESENTS

The good news is that life-practice is as easy as existing. Even better news is that there are many, many ways of doing it. In our infinite and relational universe, there is no one way of practising this life-practice; although there is only One way, which is every way.

The Universe is the sound of one hand clapping.

– Zen koan

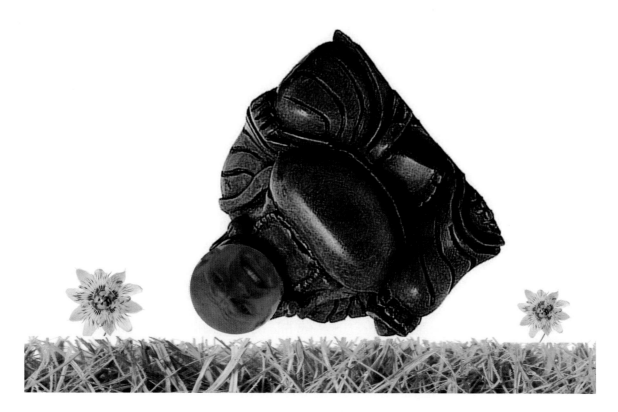

If I have given the impression at any point in this book that I am in any way even slightly competent at this stuff, you have been seriously misled. I spend most of my time falling or fallen, and very little time upright . . .

But this is a book about integrated health practice, not health theory, so let's move on. Let's start to consider how and when we are going to put some of the suggestions into practice.

When we set off on our voyage of self-discovery and self-expression, we set off on a potentially wonderful journey within which everything, and everyone, offers us a chance to learn about, and to live fully, the quite miraculous existences we have stumbled upon.

It also means living fully, despite the many, many countervailing forces that we have to face as practitioners: 'difficult' patients, traffic jams, endless targets, financial pressures, time pressures, frowning teachers, stroppy colleagues and even getting home at bath-time, hungry, grumpy and tired, to face a houseful of grumpy, tired, screaming kids.

It is possible, by applying these techniques, to pass through all the noise and chaos with perfect, balanced poise, learning, evolving and celebrating as we go.

Yeah, right.
For Buddha maybe. A tyrannical Buddha at that.

But, even for us mere mortals, this stuff can help us. The key thing is that, if we don't care properly for ourselves, we can't care properly for our patients. There are ways of caring more effectively for ourselves, as well as caring for our patients; even in real-life, full-on, poorly resourced and poorly managed healthcare systems.

FINDING INTEGRATED HARMONIC BALANCE

Healthy life practice and healthy health practice are easier if we are able to find ways that integrate all of the various entities, relationships and perspectives of our lives. These are infinite in number and scope, so we cannot hope for complete mastery of each entity, each relationship or each perspective. What we can do is to try to integrate and balance them in a way that is harmonic for us and for others, and so creates more healthy and whole existences for all of us.

Consider the analogy of the wheel. The most effective wheels are balanced, broad and smooth. There is only one place on a perfectly smoothly spinning wheel that is still, and that is the absolute centre.

Which of course (for reasons of infinite regress) cannot exist, although it must exist.

In the hectic world of health practice, trying to find our own still centres can be difficult. However, we give ourselves the best chance by making our wheel as round as possible (non-circular wheels are extremely bumpy) and as balanced as possible (spokes at different tensions will eventually crumple the wheel).

The wheel of life is therefore a very useful tool for self-assessing the balance and harmony of our lives.

'WHEEL OF LIFE' TOOLS

In the wheel of life tool (see below), each spoke corresponds to a different perspective of our existence; and the length of the each spoke corresponds to how happy we are with that area.

In the examples below we have suggested two different wheels.

1. A wheel based on the Buddhist eightfold path.
2. A wheel based on Maslow's hierarchy of needs.

Considering our lives in this way is of course only one possible perspective. It cannot capture everything. However, these wheels are useful because they remind us that our practice is part of our lives, and cannot be divorced from the rest of our lives. Therefore if we do not seek happiness and health from our practice, we will not achieve happiness and health in our lives. If we don't find happiness and health in our lives, we will not be as effective in our practice.

> There is no such thing as 'work–life' balance. Our work is our life. Our practice is our life.

Activity 9.2: The Buddhist eightfold path (30 minutes)

Thinking about your practice, mark on the wheel where you think you are in the following areas. In an area you are perfectly happy with, the spoke would reach the line of the circumference. In an area you are less happy with, it would be correspondingly shorter.

A. Seeking and finding perspective

B. Putting effort into things that further my values

C. Dedicating and committing myself to my practice

D. Living righteously

E. Becoming aware

F. Becoming mindful

G. Communicating effectively with myself

H. Acting with skill and compassion towards myself

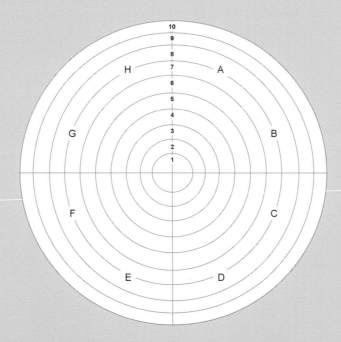

Have an honest think about how well you are caring for yourself in each of the spokes of the wheel, and consider how balanced your life may or may not be.

Activity 9.3: Maslow's hierarchy (30 minutes)

Thinking about your life practice, mark on the wheel where you think you are in the following areas. In an area you are perfectly happy with, the spoke would reach the line of the circumference. In an area you are less happy with, it would be correspondingly shorter.

A. Physiological needs

B. Safety and security needs

C. Love and belonging needs

D. Esteem needs

E. Cognitive needs

F. Aesthetic needs

G. Self-actualisation needs

H. Transcendence needs

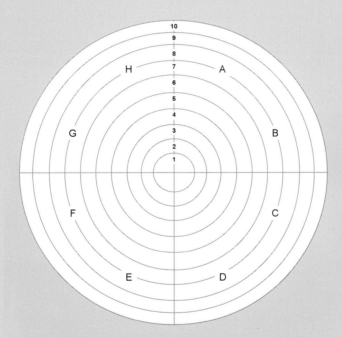

Again, have an honest think about how well you are caring for yourself in each of the spokes of the wheel, and consider how balanced your life may or may not be.

These two wheels are just examples. We can change the wheels any way we like, adding or subtracting spokes, and labelling the spokes in different ways that are more meaningful to us. For example, we could use values that are important to us, or activities that we enjoy, or dreams that we wish to fulfil. It doesn't matter. The important thing is that we choose perspectives or spokes that are important to us, here and now. Things will change, but the wheel can change with them.

PRACTISING LOVING COMPASSION WITH OURSELVES

In the rest of this series of workbooks we will move on to look at other entities in health practice, so we will take the focus off ourselves. This does not mean, however, that we should lose track of how important we are.

In these days of patient-centred practice, evidence-based practice, resource-constrained practice and outcome-led practice, we can easily forget that all practice is practitioner-founded practice. We are the foundation for all of it. Without us, there would be no patients and no health practice. Therefore we should treat ourselves as skilfully and effectively as we treat our patients.

That is easy to say and hard to do. For many reasons, some of them outlined in the preceding chapters, health practitioners often find it hard to be as caring for ourselves as we are for our patients. But we do not have to be hard on ourselves. We can take perspective.[48]

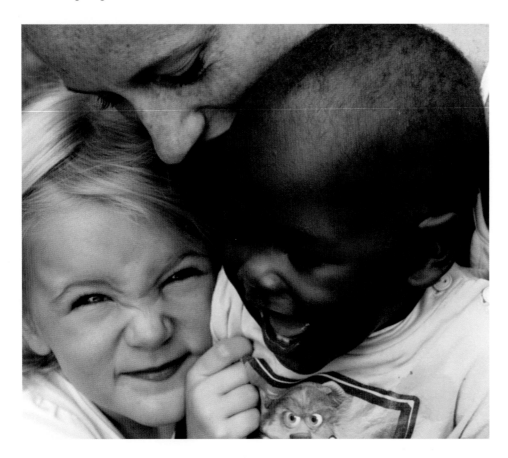

When we think about it, we are just like small children, toddling around in an enormous universe, over which we have little control and about which we have little knowledge. Just like little children, we can be selfish, ignorant and mean. But we are also like little gods, because we have the power of self-creation, and of co-creation of each other. That means we are also capable of great learning, profound trust, wondrous awareness and a deep love for everyone and everything.

It takes courage to allow this 'inner child' out. But when we do, we can start to see our lives through the eyes of that curious and inquisitive child; and we can also start to see ourselves through the eyes of a parent, with loving protection. When we err, we can correct ourselves, firmly but gently. When we fall, we can comfort ourselves and pick ourselves up. When we succeed, we can congratulate ourselves with enjoyment and pride. And at all times, we can look compassionately on ourselves and on others, with love in our hearts and a smile on our face.

Compassion

Compassion, empathy
Passion, pathos
As we feel
Our hearts daring to reveal
Then we conceive, perceive,
See with and through
Their pain and hopes
Their joys and fears
In sharing feeling
Seeing tears
We cry their pain
And then we thrill
To find our hearts being filled
With love
With lightness
From somewhere
Unknown until we dare
To open up our hearts to share
A miracle so hard to believe –
That in giving we receive.

– JA

Activity 9.4: Back to the future (at least 1 hour, hopefully every week)

Wait until no one is around, go to the playground and swing on the swings.

Really go for it. Like when you were the king (or queen) of the playground, say around 10 or 11. Old enough to impress the smaller kids, and young enough to not care what older people thought. Take it to the top, right to that point where the chain goes slack, you feel as if you will slide off, and a moment of terror grips your heart. Then feel the wonderful sense of relief and exhilaration as the chain tightens, the seat firms beneath you, and you sweep back down.

Repeat.

Many times.

Say hello to your inner child, take his (or her) hand, and allow yourself to be guided onward, to the future.

Let go of the chains, and leap. It's time to face the tyrants . . .

Notes

1 The clue is in the title. Practitioners tend to be practical. While we might like to know the theory behind what we do, what tends to be more important is that it works. The original 'Integrated Practitioner' is a whole work comprising both theory and practice. This series of workbooks is intended to be more practical, so in books 1–4 the practice will predominate. For those that are interested, the fifth workbook, *Food for Thought*, will discuss more of the theory that lies behind this work, as of course does the original book.

However, for now, please bear with us, as there are 13 key theoretical points that underpin this work and without which it may not make complete sense. They are as follows.

1. The universe, and every-'thing' within it, came into existence from no-'thing', and may presumably go back into nothing, and we can say nothing about the nothing, as there is nothing to say.

2. The universe and everything within it (including ourselves) is entirely and intrinsically relational. Within this relational web, certain states of matter and energy 'exist' (stand out) with varying degrees of complexity (entropy) against that background of nothingness.

3. Complex entities in the universe are holarchical. This means each level of complexity creates a whole which is greater than the sum of the parts. So, for example, clusters of atoms create molecules, clusters of molecules create cells, clusters of cells create organs, clusters of organs create beings, and clusters of beings create cultures and societies and biospheres. Each one of these can be said to exist on its own, as the interplay of smaller parts, and as part of the greater whole.

4. Fascinatingly, and slightly disturbingly, we find that things that may appear to us to be fixed are also relational. These include knowledge, truth, beliefs, meanings and eventually health itself. Not only are they relational, they are also self-referential. For example, truth is a function of meaning, meaning is a function of language, and language is a function of truth. Self-referential systems always end up in paradox. It is therefore impossible to define with certainty what 'health' is.

5. The universe is made up of the interplay between three things: forces, energy and matter. However, our experience of the universe is far, far richer than that. We feel warmth, beauty, taste, colour and texture. We experience anger, hope, fear, courage, joy and love. The reason that the universe appears so much richer to us is because of our consciousness. Consciousness takes in cold sense data derived from the forces, energy and matter of the universe, and uses them to

create the full richness of our existence. In other words, and in a very real way, our consciousness creates itself, and creates our experience of existence, as we go along.

6. While we think ourselves as having independent, concrete identity, this is actually just a matter of perspective. From a more macroscopic perspective, we are one infinitesimally small part of much larger relational systems: for example, our societies, our cultures, the biosphere, the noosphere, and the cosmos. From a microscopic perspective each one of our molecules and atoms comes from somewhere (or someone) else and goes somewhere (or to someone) else. From a quantum perspective we exist at the level of probability. From a cultural perspective the words, ideas and beliefs we use are mostly given to us by others.

7. When two conscious persons come into relationship with each other, each person's consciousness creates both itself and the other person. In other words, in relating to each other, in a very real way, we co-create each other.

8. Time does not flow. It is simply part of the space–time continuum. Our sense of time flowing derives from two things. First, our memory links together different states of existence in the space–time continuum in a linear way, giving us the idea that past flows into present. Second, our consciousness imagines future states of existence, giving us the idea that present flows into future.

9. This ability of consciousness to create past, present and future; to create itself; and to co-create others clearly has profound implications for what we think of as health, ill-health and health practice.

10. Health does not exist outside consciousness. It is a relational truth created by individuals, cultures and societies that has different meanings when viewed from different perspectives (for example, biomedical, psychological, sociological, or spiritual perspectives).

11. A common theme emerging from these different perspectives appears to be that health is something to do with the attainment and maintenance of a harmonic balance between different relational entities (for example, between molecules, between cells, between organs, between mind and body, between people, or between groups and societies).

12. While we cannot say what health is, we can suggest that health practice can therefore be seen as an attempt to co-create and maintain a harmonic, relational balance, not just for our patients but also for ourselves and our societies.

13. Being an integrated practitioner involves integrating all of the relationships and perspectives of our shared existence, using all of the tools that we have created and evolved through the history of human existence, to co-create 'healthier' states of existence from 'less healthy' states of existence. Health practice is therefore a science and a technology, but it is also fundamentally creative and therefore artistic.

That is enough of the theory. Let's get practical. After all, we are practitioners not theorists.

2 Edward Henry Potthast (1857–1927): 'Along the Mystic River'. Public domain art.

3 'Ars Poetica' by Archibald MacLeish, from *Collected Poems, 1917–1982*, Boston:

Houghton Mifflin; 1985. ISBN: 0395394171. Reprinted with kind permission of the Houghton Mifflin Company.

4 We seem to spend a lot of time looking for wealth and acclamation, but these do not seem to feature as sources of happiness. An interesting website to look at would be www.pursuit-of-happiness.org/history-of-happiness. Some of the key research has shown that we can learn to be happy by learning to apply our efforts in things that are important to us. The most effective of these seems to be performing acts of kindness, or when we are engaged in mindful challenges (Seligman) (what he calls 'gratifications'). Csikszentmihalyi (1997) also showed the important of the 'flow state', which is the state we enter when we are utterly absorbed by and focused on the task in hand. David Lykken and Auke Tellegen (1988) analysed thousands of middle-aged twins and found that their environmental circumstances (e.g. socioeconomic condition, religion) could account for no more than about 3% of the variance in their levels of happiness.

   We may think that money will make us happy, and to a limited extent we would be right. Once we have enough money to cover our basic needs (so we can eat, keep warm, clothe ourselves, care for the education and health of our loved ones), it appears that more money does not bring more happiness. (This is known as the Easterlin Paradox after work published in the 1970s. *See* Easterlin 1974.) It has also been more recently backed up by the Stiglitz report (Stiglitz, Sen and Fitoussi 2009) which questions the relationship between GDP and well-being.

   When we have money, it seems we do not find happiness from spending on things for ourselves, but we can find happiness on spending it on others; or on experiences with others. Outside money, happiness seems to come from loving and stable relationships; from a sense of justice; from a sense of usefulness and challenge (not too much, not too little); and from living one's life in the 'right way' (whatever that means to us).

5 Classical philosophers tended to focus on a selection of requirements for living what was called eudemonia (literally, good spirit) which was thought to closely bind up virtue, tranquillity, freedom, the absence of fear, good friendships and self-sufficiency. For Aristotle happiness rested in seeking and acting out virtue, so for him feeling well was being well: we act well because we feel well and we feel well because we act well. Judaic and Christian theologians suggested that we cannot be happy by focusing in this world, but rather that:

   'Our heart is restless until it rests in God' (Augustine).

   Whosoever trusteth in the Lord, happy is he (Proverbs 16:20)

Islamic tradition also suggests the link between happiness and righteousness:

   'Whoever does right, whether male or female, and is a believer, We will make him live a good life, and We will award them their reward for the best of what they used to do'. (Quran, 16:97).

For some traditions, this suggests a focus on the afterlife, but for mystical traditions, it may also suggest a focus on God-in-all-things.

6 The main sources of information about happiness come from ancient religions, philosophies and modern research. These suggest some common themes.

- Classical philosophy placed emphasis on living well – 'the good life' – in all senses of the word (morally, virtuously, relationally, rationally and materially).
- Psychological: the acronym PERMA has been used to describe some of the key requirements of happiness. These include the 'Pleasures' of having one's material needs met (good food, warm and safe accommodation); 'Engagement' with challenges (absorption and enjoyment of challenge, not too much but not too little either); 'Relationships' with loved ones; a sense of looking for and finding some 'Meaning'; and the satisfaction of setting and attaining some 'Accomplishments' in life.
- Biological: depression is characterised by loss of pleasure, meaning and purpose; and it can be treated with antidepressants. This suggests there is a biological element to happiness.
- Mystical teachings suggest some form of perspective gained by placing one's life in the context of the vastness of everything; some form of renunciation of egoistic and selfish drives; and forming and practising loving compassion.
- Economic: economic research suggests a basic level of wealth is necessary for happiness; as is a relative equality between richer and poorer people in our societies. Significant wealth, however, does not seem to be a key factor behind happiness.

7 A report presented to the Foresight Project on communicating the evidence base for improving people's well-being, written by: Jody Aked, Nic Marks, Corrina Cordon, Sam Thompson, published by the Centre for Well-being, NEF (the New Economics Foundation) is an excellent review of the evidence on happiness, and well worth reading (*see* Aked *et al.* 2008). The authors conclude that there are five things we can do to find more happiness:

- connecting with as many people as possible in a friendly and loving way
- being active
- being mindful and aware
- keep learning and keep challenging yourself
- giving compassionately to other people.

8 From the report *Mental Capital and Wellbeing: making the most of ourselves in the 21st century* by the Foresight Project, 2008. Reprinted with kind permission of the Foresight Project.

9 The Buddhist eightfold path fundamentally aims to free its practitioners from suffering, by pointing out and seeking freedom from the illusions, distractions and attachments that we, as self-conscious and creative beings, find all too easy to create and then attach to. Buddhism teaches four fundamental tenets (what it calls 'Noble Truths'). These are that:

- suffering is inherent for all sentient beings
- we suffer because we get attached to and crave things that are impermanent and which inevitably decay and corrupt
- we can cease suffering by removing our attachment to impermanent and transient things

- we can find a way to achieve cessation of suffering which is reasonable and avoids the extremes of hedonism and asceticism by taking a particular path that gradually helps us to dissipate craving and ignorance (the eightfold path).

The eight steps on the path are as follows.

- Right View: recognising that everything is relational, imperfect and impermanent (including ourselves). This 'right view' helps us put, and keep, things in proper perspectives, rather than striving for and attaching ourselves to things that are worthless.
- Right Intention: making the decision, not just once but continuously, to dedicate and commit ourselves to living more ethically and effectively.
- Right Speech: abstain from lying or deception, abstaining from using unkind or hurtful speech, and using speech for effective and worthwhile purposes rather than for inane or idle chatter.
- Right Action: being non-violent, honest, charitable and faithful to others.
- Right Livelihood: trying to choose and live a life that is righteous in its aims and outcomes.
- Right Effort: using our energy to try to bring about wholesome and worthwhile aims (such as kindness, benevolence and constructiveness) rather than unwholesome ones (such as violence, anger, aggression, envy and lust).
- Right Mindfulness: training ourselves to see and experience things as they are, in the here and now, rather than getting sucked into an internal morass of anxiety, rumination, emotion and false impression.
- Right Concentration: attempting to channel our minds and focus on one single point at a time, so we unify and direct our energies most effectively and efficiently, developing and building concentration.

10 Mindfulness is a form of self-awareness training adapted from mindfulness meditation. Mindfulness is about being aware of what is happening in the present on a moment by moment basis, while not making judgements about whether we like or don't like what we find.

11 'Complete Happiness' by Bonnie Lanzillotta, which was hung in the Massachusetts General Cancer Center in Boston, MA; 2011. More of Bonnie's work can be found at www.bonnielanzillotta.com. The image is reproduced with kind permission of the artist, who maintains copyright.

12 Psychologists suggest that the pursuit of happiness seems to be possible as long as it is carried out wisely. We have to say 'wisely' because we seem to be very poor predictors of what it is that will make us happy or unhappy. We seem to be able to recover from extremes of happiness and unhappiness (such as winning the lottery or losing one's legs) in a way that we do not predict (*see* David Gilbert, *Stumbling on Happiness*. New York: Vintage; 2007). In other words, we seem to have a baseline state of happiness to which we are able to find our way back after such events.

This baseline state of happiness seems to come from a number of sources. Our overall approach to life seems important. If we can approach it with equanimity (keeping a broader sense of perspective), being optimistic (seeing the glass as half full), staying healthy (eating, sleeping and exercising well), and making time for fun as well as for work, we will stand a much better chance of being happy.

13 Most theories recognise the particular importance of the 'critical learning period', which are the first three to four years of our lives, during which we lay down attitudes towards and perspectives of ourselves, others and the world around us. During the first few years our brains are still 'plastic' and able to rewire themselves. After this period, while we can still teach old dogs new tricks, it seems to be much harder to change fundamental attitudes. *See* the chapter 'Playing' in workbook 2 for more details.

14 'Vanishing Venice' (2007), oil on board, by Patrick Hughes. The image has been reproduced with kind permission of the artist. More of Patrick's work in art, perspective and paradox can be seen at www.patrickhughes.co.uk

15 There are many, many theories about personality types and traits, but we will just deal with a few of the major ones here. Concepts of introversion and extraversion have been around for centuries; and the oldest personality theories were based on the idea that our personalities derive from the balance of 'four elements' (fire, water, earth and air) relating to 'four humours' (blood, phlegm, yellow bile and black bile). Jung also believed that there are four main personality types: thinking, feeling, sensing and intuition. This theory was built upon by Myers and Briggs to create the well-known Myers Briggs Inventory, which in turn led to Keirsey's typologies. Freud's theory was that the personality is due to the interplay of three significant components: the id (focusing on pleasure and satisfaction of desires), the ego (focusing on practicality, organisation and rationality) and the super-ego (focusing on conscience and morality). Eysenck believed that there are two major dimensions, balancing in different ways: introversion–extraversion and stability–instability.

   The theories above are psychodynamic, in that they are interior interpretations of existence. Psychologists last century attempted to approach personality scientifically, and studies have consistently suggested five major personality dimensions (termed the 'Big Five' by Goldberg: *see* Goldberg 1993) and commonly referred to as the OCEAN model. These are Openness to experience (balanced between 'creative' and 'conforming'); Conscientiousness (balanced between detailed and unstructured); Extraversion (balanced with introversion); Agreeableness (balanced with tough-mindedness) and Neuroticism (balanced between self-confidence and sensitivity).

   If you want to have a look at how some of these work with your own personality try the following.
   • For your big five typology go to http://test.personality-project.org
   • For a free Jungian/Myers Briggs related typology, try www.humanmetrics.com (if you want the full Myers Briggs you need to pay for formal testing).
   • For your Keirsey temperament try www.keirsey.com

16 Original article by: Henning *et al.* 1998.

17 Many philosophies and religions have value systems that we may ascribe to, such as the following.
   • Christian and Judaic values might be captured by (Dt 6:4): 'Hear, O Israel, the Lord our God is one Lord; and you shall love the Lord your God with all your heart, and with all your soul, and with all your might' and Lv 19:18 'You shall love your neighbour as yourself'.
   • Islamic values might be captured by this passage from the Quran (2:177): 'It is

not righteousness that you turn your faces towards the East or West; but it is righteousness to believe in God and the Last Day and the Angels, and the Book, and the Messengers; to spend of your substance, out of love for Him, for your kin, for orphans, for the needy, for the wayfarer, for those who ask, and for the freeing of captives; to be steadfast in prayers, and practise regular charity; to fulfil the contracts which you made; and to be firm and patient in pain and adversity and throughout all periods of panic. Such are the people of truth, the God-conscious.'

- Catholics have suggested that there are seven virtues: the four cardinal virtues of prudence, justice, restraint, and courage, and the three theological virtues of faith, hope, and love.

- Buddhists suggest: 'The greatest achievement is selflessness. The greatest worth is self-mastery. The greatest quality is seeking to serve others. The greatest precept is continual awareness. The greatest medicine is the emptiness of everything. The greatest action is not conforming with the world's ways. The greatest magic is transmuting the passions. The greatest generosity is non-attachment. The greatest goodness is a peaceful mind. The greatest patience is humility. The greatest effort is not concerned with results. The greatest meditation is a mind that lets go. The greatest wisdom is seeing through appearances.' Atisha (11th-century Tibetan Buddhist master)

- Kant suggested a universal moral law which he described as the 'categorical imperative': Act in such a way that you treat humanity, whether in your own person or in the person of any other, never merely as a means to an end, but always at the same time as an end.' (Immanuel Kant, *Groundwork of the Metaphysic of Morals; see* Kant 2002).

18 Stress is a syndrome of over-engagement when we become urgent and over-reactive (even hyperactive). We may lack concentration, have poor timekeeping, poor productivity and difficulty in comprehending new procedures. We might become uncooperative, irritable or aggressive. Importantly for our work, we start to lose compassion and start to make mistakes.

Ultimately, if stress continues beyond our ability to cope, we might begin to burn out. Unlike stress, which is a syndrome of mental and physical over-engagement, burnout is more characterised by under-engagement: mental and physical withdrawal and shut-down. Burnout reduces our productivity and saps our energy, leaving us feeling increasingly hopeless, powerless, cynical and resentful.

Usually, the first people to notice when someone is burning out are family and friends. Later, we tend to give up trying to hide it at work, and the problems become apparent to colleagues. Usually, we avoid showing signs to patients until the effects are advanced.

19 According to Maslach *et al.* (2001), burnout is the degree of 'dislocation between what people are and what they have to do'. It is a syndrome of emotional exhaustion, depersonalisation, low productivity, and feelings of low achievement. Although it can occur in a range of occupations, burnout has been found to occur most among professional people in the caring professions of medicine, nursing, social work, counselling and teaching. It manifests itself in the form of chronic exhaustion, cynical detachment, and feelings of ineffectiveness. Burnout reduces our productivity

and saps our energy, leaving us feeling increasingly hopeless, powerless, cynical and resentful.

Practitioners who are stressed or burnt out usually are able to hide this from patients until quite late on (and well after they start affecting interpersonal and team relationships at work). Nevertheless, ultimately patient care will begin to suffer and effects can include: making mistakes, poor time-keeping, sickness, loss of patience, loss of empathy, inability to listen fully to patient concerns, and poor communication with colleagues.

Negative effects of burnout in practice include the following:
- poor patient compliance (DiMatteo *et al.* 1993)
- poor patient satisfaction (Linn *et al.* 1985)
- riskier prescribing profiles (Melville 1980)
- mental health problems and suicide (Arnetz & Horte 1987)
- disruption of work performance, including absenteeism, job turnover, poor job performance, accidents and errors, and alcohol and drug abuse, documented in a recent review of the general stress literature (Kahn & Byosiere 1992)
- increased job turnover (Buchbinder *et al.* 1999)
- physical ill health (Lazarus & Folkman 1984)
- reduced performance and absenteeism (Ivancevich & Matteson 1980).

20 Factors that affect resilience, coping and burnout include (adapted from Amery 2009 for more details) include the following.
- Age: the word 'burnout' suggests a time factor is important – that the longer we work the more likely we are to burn out. In fact (counter-intuitively) the highest risk of burnout tends to occur in the first 2–3 years of a new job. Probably, as we get older, we learn more about ourselves and learn stronger and better ways of coping, or simply move on to another job where we feel more comfortable.
- Health and energy: if we eat well, sleep well and exercise well, we keep ourselves fit and energetic. If we are fit and energetic, we are much better able to resist the pressures of our work.
- Positive belief (e.g. optimism): those who see the glass as half full rather than half empty seem to be more resilient. It is not easy to change the way we look at the world, but we can try to see the best rather than the worst in things.
- Problem-solving skills: people who are able to break problems down into chunks small enough to tackle, and then plan how to face these problems, tend to be more resilient. If you are not like this, try to speak to people who are, share your issue and learn from them as they assist you in solving problems.
- Social skills: people who have better social skills are better at winning people round to their way of thinking, recruiting people to their cause, and motivating others to stay with them. You may not have ideal social skills, but they can be improved through getting feedback, advice and coaching from colleagues.
- Assertiveness: we all need to be able to say no to the demands placed on us. There is more suffering and there are more patients in the world than any of us can possibly help with. Demands are endless and at times overwhelming. Those who can remember their own needs among the crush of those of their patients are better able to cope.

- Resources: if you don't have enough money, or time, or help from others, it goes without saying that you will struggle more than people who do. You might not be able to do much about your personal circumstances, but you can choose which problems you can realistically take on with the resources that you do have.
- Degree of personal control: if you feel out of control, it is natural to be fearful, and fear weakens our resolve. You might be stuck in your situation, but often there are ways out, either by trying to tackle the problem or to walk away from it altogether. A job is just that: a job. It's not worth losing your health over.
- Being unmarried or not having children: being married and having children seem to be protective (again counter-intuitively to those of us who feel at wits' end coping with our families!).
- Caring for others at home: people who care for others at home (not surprisingly) tend to have higher rates of burnout than those who don't.
- Social support: being lonely is a major cause of unhappiness; and people who are lonely have fewer sources of support and also fewer people to distract them and share their problem.
- Work overload: every individual and every team has a limit to what they can do in the time allocated. Even the most efficient and effective team will get exhausted eventually. Good managers need to limit overtime and on-call, ensure adequate meal breaks, and discourage 'stay-late' syndrome (which is very common in the 'superman/wonderwoman' care type). Health practice is not regular: there are peaks and troughs of activity. Management needs to plan not just for the average workload but also for the extremes, and build in sufficient tolerance.
- Role clarity: when team members' individual roles are not clear, or not understood, or blurred, conflicts and burnout are more likely to arise. We need to know the limits of our job if we are to set boundaries. Without clear boundaries, we cannot plan our time or energies properly.
- Home–work boundaries: like role clarity, we need to know how long we are to be at work, when we can go off, and when we have to be on-call, so that we can plan our resources.
- Fear of job loss, discipline, bullying or other abuse at work: managers need to take care to create a supportive, non-abusive and encouraging environment. High-blame environments do not support good practice.
- Change: high rates of staff turnover, frequent policy changes, and other changes are unsettling. We should also remember that resistance to change is a feature of early burnout. The combination of the two means that managers have to take great care introducing and implanting change, ensuring that change is agreed with the team and that it is introduced within the abilities of the team to absorb it.
- Unrealistic goals: teams, like individuals, can set themselves unrealistic goals. Mangers also can expect too much. Good managers recognise the capacity of their team, build in some tolerance, and only allow their teams to fight battles they have a realistic chance of winning. Teams and individuals need some challenge, but not too much either.

21 The practice of applying morals or values to our choices and actions is ethics. Underlying most ethics is the attempt to decide whether a particular choice or

particular action actualises a new present which avoids breaking the values, beliefs and laws of the persons and cultures involved.

22 *See* Chapter 6, Becoming Aware and Mindful, for more information on the 'flow' state.

23 In a 2003 study Firth-Cozens (2003) assessed people hospitalised for depression for their degree of perfectionism, hopelessness and negative cognitive bias. Perfectionism was shown to be an excellent predictor for a patient's suicidal ideation six months after hospitalisation, shattering the common notion that hopelessness is the best warning sign of future suicidal thoughts.

24 Perfectionism can be seen as a form of low self esteem, with denial defences built around it. It can be compounded by health practitioner training where teaching can often be demanding, critical and undermining. The combination of low self esteem, denial and perfectionism can be viewed as a form of narcissism: 'I don't make mistakes, I'm perfect.' The splitting that this causes is exhausting; it can easily spill over into arrogance and inability to receive or learn from criticism.

25 Named by after Pareto (an economist) who observed that 80% of the land in Italy was owned by 20% of the population. This principle was first applied by Juran in the 1940s (*see* Juran & Gryna 1988) to economics, but it has been applied successfully in economics, business and computing. Further information can be found in Koch (2001).

26 Ketut is the Balinese healer described in *Eat, Pray, Love: one woman's search for everything* by Elizabeth Gilbert (*see* Gilbert 2006).

27 This is an ancient Balinese sacred picture which was shown in the film *Eat, Pray, Love* by Ketut, the Balinese healer consulted by the author, who was trying to find some peace in her life.

28 Image reproduced under licence from www.photos.com

29 Mindfulness is a form of self-awareness training adapted from mindfulness meditation. Mindfulness is about being aware of what is happening in the present on a moment by moment basis, while not making judgements about whether we like or don't like what we find.

We all have the capacity to be mindful. It simply involves cultivating our ability to pay attention in the present moment and allows us to disengage from mental 'clutter' and to have a clear mind. It makes it possible for us to respond rather than react to situations, thus improving our decision making and potential for physical and mental relaxation.

It is not simply a relaxation technique or 'power of positive thinking'. The technique is based on Buddhist meditation principles but was described by Teasdale (*see* Segal, Williams & Teasdale 2001) and Beck for use in treatment of depression and then used by Linehan as a core skill in her cognitive behavioural therapy for borderline personality disorder. Linehan (1993) describes:

- three 'what' skills: observing (simply attending to events and emotions), describing (applying labels to behaviours, emotions and situations) and participating (entering into current activities)
- three 'how' skills: taking a 'non-judgemental' stance, focusing on one thing in the moment and being effective (doing what is needed rather than worrying about what is right or second guessing the situation).

30 From *Buddha's Little Instruction Book*. (Kornfield 1996).

31 Csikszentmihalyi & Nakamura, The concept of flow, in *Handbook of Positive Psychology* (Snyder and Lopez 2002), pp. 89–92.

32 Csikszentmihalyi (1997).

33 Image from www.Gettyimages.com

34 Health practitioners have higher levels of mental ill health than the general population. Some 25% of UK doctors are suffering with depression or anxiety at any one time. If you add alcoholism and other substance abuse, the figure is even higher (a report from the BMA in the UK stated that over 7% of doctors were addicted to alcohol or other chemical substances, and that 23% of GPs had increased their drinking in response to stress). Health practitioners have higher levels of alcoholism, depression, drug misuse and suicide than average and the highest incidence of work-related mental ill health than any profession except the army. Mental ill health seems to be caused by workload, inadequate resources, poor support, high demand, dealing with suffering, poor relationships, poor team working, regulations and investigations, complaints, and the competing tensions of work and home life. Furthermore, most of us are dealing with significant organisational and cultural change in the workplace. This includes: multidisciplinary working, greater scrutiny and criticism of professions, critical enquiries, patients being more likely to challenge their practitioners' views, and the sense of loss of autonomy and control but with a continuing sense that the 'buck stops with me'.

35 There are a number of inventories online. Try the Black Dog Institute website www.blackdoginstitute.org.au

36 There are some excellent resources for practitioners with mental health problems at the Black Dog Institute website (www.blackdoginstitute.org.au). The following texts may also be useful: Kabat-Zinn (1991), Brantley (2007), Linehan (1993), McQuaid & Carmona (2004), Segal, Williams & Teasdale (2001), Thich Nhat Hanh, Mobi Ho, Vo-Dinh Mai (1975).

37 One minute exercise: sit in front of a clock, let your body drop into softness and relaxation, and simply feel your breath gently flowing in and out. Choose one place to feel your breath flowing; e.g. at the tip of your nose, the back of the throat, or the depth of your lungs.

Awareness exercise: take an erect and dignified posture. Then ask yourself: 'What is going on with me at the moment?' Simply allow yourself to observe whatever happens. Label any thoughts that you have and then leave them alone. Don't engage with them but just let them float away. Attend to your breathing or simply take in your surroundings instead. Besides thoughts, there may be sounds you hear, bodily sensations that you are aware of. If you find yourself constantly elaborating on thoughts, rather than labelling them and returning to the neutral, remember to observe your breathing. When emotions or memories of painful events occur, don't allow yourself to become caught up by them. Give them short labels such as 'that's a sad feeling', 'that's an angry feeling' and then just allow them to drift or float away. These memories and feelings will gradually decrease in intensity and frequency.

If you have difficulty not engaging with thoughts or emotions, you can use techniques for blocking them. A visual technique is to imagine a black box with a big lock. Visualise unwanted thoughts disappearing into the box and being locked away. An auditory technique is to choose a word or phrase to repeat every time a thought becomes intrusive, for example 'peace' or 'watching' or 'letting go'.

Mindful eating: when you next eat, try to set aside any distractions. If you have kids, bad luck. Perhaps you can see them as a welcome opportunity to learn even greater patience! Pay full attention to what you eat: the look of the food, the colour of the plate, the contrasts of textures and colours, the smells before you taste, your mouth tingling in anticipation, the feel and temperature of the food in the front, then back of your mouth, the sensation when you swallow, and the warm feeling of repleteness as you finish.

Mindful walking: concentrate on the feel of the ground under your feet, your breathing while walking. Just observe what is around you as you walk, staying in the present. Let your other thoughts go, just look at the sky, the view, the other walkers; feel the wind, the temperature on your skin; enjoy the moment.

As you become more practised at mindfulness, you will become more aware of yourself as an 'outside observer' or 'witness' rather than a person who is disturbed by these thoughts and feelings. By obtaining and holding a more non-attached perspective, it is easier to stay calm and focus and choose more effective and efficient courses of action, which is very useful in health practice.

38 Some 'self' theories suggests our minds are actually 'societies' of many voices and positions all of which are in dialogue with each other. Wisdom teachings have described the self as many selves for thousands of years. In modern times, in 1950, William James (James 2010) drew attention to the distinction between the self as subject (the 'I') and the self as object (the 'Me'). In 1993, in Dialogical Self Theory, Hermans *et al.* (Hermans & Kempen 1993, Hermans & Gieser 2011) extended the concept even further, pointing out that not only does the self contain a number of different perspectives and positions 'internally', the self also projects itself 'externally' into our outer relationships. Thus the boundary between where the 'self' begins and ends, and where the 'other' begins and ends, is extremely blurry and leaky. We 'import' parts of the other into ourselves and 'export' parts of ourselves into the other. We can hear this in phrases such as 'I would have but I could hear him telling me not to'. That is why we can experience such things as self-conflict and self-criticism, and use reflexive speech. By becoming aware of all these different 'selves' we can prevent some becoming tyrannical, and use the 'internal dialogue' as a means for personal development and growth.

39 When we think of ourselves we tend to do so by assessing and then categorising ourselves. We then start to 'know' ourselves by these different labels. These labels might include, for example, father, introvert, doctor, bald, football fan, caring, emotional and so on. Our self-concept is in a constant state of flux as different experiences lead to different self-assessments and self-categorisations. However, there are some self-concepts that we may have difficulty accepting, even despite evidence to the contrary. For example, bullies may have no self-concept of themselves as 'bullies' but might accept a 'physical' or 'expressive' or even 'short-tempered' self-concept. When we are faced with very difficult self-concepts (for example: as a victim, or as

weak, or as imperfect) we may split these off entirely, so they disappear out of direct consciousness, to lurk in our subconscious, either latently or destructively.

40 Splitting is the term used when we find it difficult or impossible to integrate aspects of ourselves into a unified and coherent whole. It often results from defence mechanisms, where unwelcome or unwanted positions, beliefs or emotions are separated out and cut off from the conscious. It was first described by Pierre Janet and Sigmund Freud, and later developed by Melanie Klein.

41 Our self narratives help us to develop our identity, and may indeed be at the heart of what the self actually is. In health practice, narratives are very important in that they help us make sense of new (and unpleasant) illness realities, and can be used by the practitioner to develop more healthy self-concepts and outcomes (*see* the chapter 'Storytelling' in workbook 2 for more details).

42 Psychodrama is not dissimilar to narrative theory, but puts the emphasis more on how internal narratives and beliefs are acted out in practice. It can also be used as a tool for diagnosis and management in practice. *See* the chapter 'Acting' in workbook 2 for more details.

43 Carl Jung used the term 'wounded healer' to describe the way that practitioners draw on their own experiences of pain and suffering to develop empathic understanding and relationship with our patients. Rather than seeing our internal conflicts and pains as an obstacle to be overcome in order to be able to practise objectively, Jung fully embraced the subjectivity of practice, and viewed it as an effective tool to be used. For more information, *see* the chapter 'Transferring and counter transferring' in workbook 2.

44 *See*, e.g. Eve 2003.

45 Maslow's theory first appeared in a 1943 paper: 'A theory of human motivation' (Maslow 1943).

46 1969 article, 'Theory Z' (reprinted in Maslow's basic text on Transpersonal Psychology, *The Farther Reaches of Human Nature*, *see* Maslow 1976).

47 'Transcend Conformity' by Sara Ann Zimmerman, reproduced with kind permission of the author. More of Sara's work can be seen at http://fineartamerica.com/profiles/sara-ann-zimmerman.html

48 There are now many tools that we can use to get an objective assessment of where we are, and that can help us take perspective. Some useful tools (and websites) are as follows.
- Interview yourself
- The burnout inventory
- Depression inventory
- Anxiety inventory
- Substance abuse
- Job satisfaction inventory
- Attributional Style Questionnaire (ASQ)
- Curiosity and Exploration Inventory (CEI)
- Gratitude Questionnaire – 6 (GQ-6)
- Hope Scale (HS)
- Inspiration Scale (IS)

- Meaning in Life Questionnaire (MLQ)
- Mindful Attention Awareness Scale (MAAS)
- Older Adults' Attributional Style Questionnaire (OAASQ)
- Personal Growth Initiative Scale (PGIS)
- Psychological Well-Being Scales
- Quality of Life Inventory (QOLI)
- Satisfaction with Life Scale
- Silver Lining Questionnaire (SLQ)
- State-Trait-Cheerfulness Inventory (STCI)
- Subjective Happiness Scale (SHS)
- Transgression-Related Interpersonal Motivations Inventory (TRIM)
- VIA Inventory of Strengths (VIA-IS).

All of these can be found at 'Open Door Coaching' at www.opendoorcoaching.com. Copyright © 2003 Marcia Bench And Career Coach Institute; Reprinted With Permission.

Bibliography

Abbasi K. Doctors: automatons, technicians, or knowledge brokers? *JRSM*. 2007; **100**(1): 1. Print.

Aked J, Marks N, Cordon C, Thompson S. Five ways to well-being. *Foresight Project on Mental Capital and Wellbeing*. New Economics Foundation; 2008. Web. Available at: www.neweconomics.org/publications/five-ways-well-being-evidence

Alladin A, Alibhai A. Cognitive hypnotherapy for depression: an empirical investigation. *IJCEH*. 2007; **55**(2): 147–66. Print.

Allen RP. *Scripts and Strategies in Hypnotherapy: the complete works*. Carmarthen: Crown House Publishing; 2004. Print.

Ambady N. Surgeons' tone of voice: a clue to malpractice history. *Surgery*. 2002; **132**(1): 5–9. Print.

Amery J. *Children's Palliative Care in Africa*. Oxford: Oxford University Press; 2009. Print.

Anielski M. *The Economics of Happiness: building genuine wealth*. Gabriola, BC: New Society; 2007. Print.

Armstrong D. Space and time in British general practice. *Soc Sci Med*. 1985; **20**(7): 659–66. Print.

Arnetz BB, Horte LG. Suicide patterns among physicians related to other academics as well as to the general populations: results from a national long-term prospective study and a retrospective study. *Acta Psychiatr Scand*. 1987; **75**(2): 139–43. Print.

Balint M. *The Doctor, His Patient, and the Illness*. New York: International Universities; 1957. Print.

Bandura A. Self-efficacy: toward a unifying theory of behavioral change. *Psychol Rev*. 1977; **84**(2): 191–215. Print.

Barsky AJ. Hidden reasons some patients visit doctors. *Ann Intern Med*. 1981; **94**: 492–8. Print.

Beating the Blues®. Web. Available at: www.beatingtheblues.co.uk (accessed 28 October 2011).

Beck DE, Cowan CC. *Spiral Dynamics*. Oxford: Blackwell; 2006. Print.

Beckman HB, Frankel RM. The effect of physician behavior on the collection of data. *Ann Intern Med*. 1984; **101**: 692–6. Print.

Beevers CG, Miller IW. Perfectionism, cognitive bias, and hopelessness as prospective predictors of suicidal ideation. *Suicide and Life-Threatening Behavior*. 2004; **34**(2): 126–37. Print.

Bench M. Open Door Coaching. Web. Available at: www.opendoorcoaching.com. (accessed 17 October 2011). Copyright © 2003 Marcia Bench and Career Coach Institute; reprinted with permission.

Berne E. *Games People Play: the psychology of human relationships*. New York: Grove; 1964. Print.

Betancourt JR, Ananeh-Firempong O. Not me! Doctors, decisions, and disparities in health care: how do we really make decisions? *Cardiovasc Rev Rep.* 2004; **25**(3): n.p. Print.

Better Health. Web. Available at: http://getbetterhealth.com (accessed 17 October 2011).

Black Dog Institute. *Depression.* Black Dog Institute. Web. Available at: www.black doginstitute.org.au (accessed 23 November 2011).

Blanck PD, Buck R, Rosenthal R. *Nonverbal Communication in the Clinical Context.* University Park: Pennsylvania State University Press; 1986. Print.

Blenkiron P. *Stories and Analogies in Cognitive Behavioural Therapy.* Oxford: Wiley Blackwell; 2010. Print.

Block N. How many concepts of consciousness? *Behavioral and Brain Sciences.* 1995; **18**(2):272–8. Print.

BMJ. How much do we know? Clinical Evidence. BMJ. Web. Available at: http://clinical evidence.bmj.com/ceweb/about/knowledge.jsp (accessed 17 October 2011)

Bohm D. *Wholeness and the Implicate Order.* London: Routledge & Kegan Paul; 1981. Print.

Bradford VTS. Trainers' Toolkit. Home. Web. Available at: www.bradfordvts.co.uk (accessed 12 November 2011).

Brantley J. *Calming Your Anxious Mind: how mindfulness and compassion can free you from anxiety, fear, and panic.* Oakland, CA: New Harbinger Publications; 2007. Print.

British Association for Behavioural & Cognitive Psychotherapies. Home Page. Web. Available at: www.babcp.com (accessed 28 October 2011).

British Medical Association. *Doctors' Health.* 8 May 2007. Web. Available at: www.bma. org.uk/doctors_health/doctorshealth.jsp?page=2 (accessed 28 October 2011).

British Medical Association. *Quality and Outcomes Framework, February 2010.* Web. Available at: www.bma.org.uk/employmentandcontracts/independent_contractors/ quality_outcomes_framework/qualityframework10.jsp (accessed 28 October 2011).

Brown D. Evidence-based hypnotherapy for asthma: a critical review. *IJCEH.* 2007; **55**(2): 220–49. Print.

Bruton HJ. Book review: nations and households in economic growth: essays in honor of Moses Abramovitz (Paul A. David, Melvin W. Reder). *Economic Development and Cultural Change.* 1979; **27**(4): 801. Print.

Bstan-'dzin-rgya-mtsho, Hopkins J. *Becoming Enlightened.* New York: Atria; 2009. Print.

Buber M. *I and Thou.* New York: Continuum; 2004. Print.

Buchbinder SB, Wilson M, Melick CF. Estimates of costs of primary care physician turnover. *Am J Managed Care.* 1999; **5**(11): 1431. Print.

Businessballs. *Job Satisfaction Inventory.* Businessballs Free Online Learning for Careers, Work, Management, Business Training and Education. Web. Available at: http:// businessballs.com (accessed 27 October 2011).

Businessballs. Web. Available at: http://businessballs.com (accessed 24 October 2011).

Byrne PS, Long BEL. *Doctors Talking to Patients.* London: HMSO; 1978. Print.

Campbell DT. Blind variation and selective retention in creative thought as in other knowledge processes. *Psychol Rev.* 1960; **67**: 380–400. Print.

Campling P, Haigh R. *Therapeutic Communities: past, present, and future.* London: Jessica Kingsley; 1999. Print.

Campo R. What the body told. *The World in Us: lesbian and gay poetry of the next wave.* New York: Griffin; 2001. N.p. Print.

Caplan F, Caplan T. *The Power of Play.* New York: Doubleday; 1973. Print.

Carroll L, Green RL. *Alice's Adventures in Wonderland; and, through the looking-glass and what Alice found there.* London: Oxford University Press; 1971. Print.

Casey PR, Tyrer P. Personality disorder and psychiatric illness in general practice. *Br J Psychiatry.* 1990; **156**(2): 261–5. Print.

Chomsky N. A minimalist program for linguistic theory. *The View from the Building: essays in honor of Sylvain Bromberger.* Cambridge: MIT; 1993. N.p. Print.

Cole SA, Bird J. *The Medical Interview: the three-function approach.* St. Louis: Mosby; 2000. Print.

Committee on the Use of Complementary and Alternative Medicine by the American Public. *Complementary and Alternative Medicine in the United States.* Washington, DC: National Academies; 2005. Print.

Covey, S. *The 7 Habits Of Highly Effective People.* Free Press; Revised edition 2004.

Cozens J. Doctors, their wellbeing and stress. *BMJ.* 2003; **326**: 670–1. Print.

Csikszentmihalyi M. *Finding Flow: the psychology of engagement with everyday life.* New York: Basic; 1997. Print.

Dalai Lama. *Becoming Enlightened.* London: Rider; 2010. Print.

Dalai Lama, Cutler HC. *The Art of Happiness: a handbook for living.* Audiobook CD. New York: Simon & Schuster Audio; 1998.

Dalai Lama, Hopkins J. *Becoming Enlightened.* New York: Atria; 2009. Print.

Damgaard-Mørch NL, Nielsen LJ, Uldwall SW. [Knowledge and perceptions of complementary and alternative medicine among medical students in Copenhagen]. [Article in Danish] Ugeskr Laeger. 2008; **170**(48): 3941–5. Available in translation at: www.vifab.dk/uk/statistics/medical+students+and+alternative+medicine?

Davison S. Principles of managing patients with personality disorder. *Adv Psychiatr Treat.* 2002; **8**: 1–9. Print.

Deber RB. What role do patients wish to play in treatment decision making? *Arch Intern Med.* 1996; **156**: 1414–20. Print.

de Girolamo G, Reich JH. *Epidemiology of Mental Disorders and Psychosocial Problems: personality disorders.* Geneva: World Health Organization; 1993. Print.

DeLongis A, Folkman S, Lazarus RS. The impact of daily stress on health and mood: psychological and social resources as mediators. *J Pers Soc Psychol.* 1988; **54**(3): 486–95. Print.

Dennett DC. *Consciousness Explained.* London: Penguin; 1993. Print.

Deveugele M, Derese A, van den Brink-Muinen A, *et al.* Consultation length in general practice: cross sectional study in six European countries. *BMJ.* 2002; **325**(7362): 472. Print.

Dewey J. *How We Think.* Boston: D.C. Heath & Co; 1910. Print.

Dickinson E, Franklin RW. *The Poems of Emily Dickinson*. Cambridge, MA: Belknap of Harvard University Press; 1998. Print.

Digman JM. Personality structure: emergence of the five-factor model. *Annu Rev Psychology*. 1990; **41**(1): 417–40. Print.

DiMatteo M, Robin CD, Sherbourne RD, *et al*. Physicians' characteristics influence patients' adherence to medical treatment: results from the Medical Outcomes Study. *Health Psychol*. 1993; **12**(2): 93–102. Print.

DOH. *Improving Access to Psychological Therapies (IAPT) Programme: computerised Cognitive Behavioural Therapy (cCBT) implementation guidance*. Department of Health, UK; March 2007. Web. Available at: www.dh.gov.uk/en/Publicationsand statistics/Publications/PublicationsPolicyAndGuidance/DH_073470

DOH. *Delivering Care, Improving Outcomes for Patients*. Quality and Outcomes Framework; 8 February 2010.

DOH. *Mental Health and Ill Health in Doctors*. London: Crown Publishing; 2008. Department of Health. Web. Available at: www.dh.gov.uk/en/Publicationsandstatistics/ Publications/PublicationsPolicyAndGuidance/DH_083066.

DOH. *Mental Health Policy Implementation Guide: adult acute inpatient care provision*. Department of Health (UK); 2002. Web. Available at: www.positive-options.com/ news/downloads/DoH_-_Adult_Acute_In-patient_Care_Provision_-_2002.pdf.

DOH. *The GP Patient Survey: general information*. The GP Patient Survey. UK Department of Health; 2010. Web. Available at: www.gp-patient.co.uk/info

Doran T. Effect of financial incentives on incentivised and non-incentivised clinical activities: longitudinal analysis of data from the UK Quality and Outcomes Framework. *BMJ*. 2011; **342**: 590–8. Print.

Dowson JH, Grounds A. *Personality Disorders: recognition and clinical management*. Cambridge: Cambridge University Press; 1995. Print.

Dunnette MD, Hough LM, Triandis HC. *Handbook of Industrial and Organizational Psychology*. Palo Alto, CA: Consulting Psychologists; 1990. Print.

Durkheim É, Cladis CS. *The Elementary Forms of Religious Life*. Oxford: Oxford University Press; 2001. Print.

Durojave OC. Health screening: is it always worth doing? *The Internet Journal of Epidemiology*. 2009; **7**(1): n.p. Print.

Easterlin RA. Does economic growth improve the human lot? Some empirical evidence. In: David PA, Reder MW, editors. *Nations and Households in Economic Growth: essays in honor of Moses Abramovitz*. New York: Academic Press; 1974. Print.

Edelman GM, Mountcastle VB. *The Mindful Brain: cortical organization and the group-selective theory of higher brain function*. Cambridge: MIT; 1978. Print.

Edelman GM, Tononi G. *A Universe of Consciousness: how matter becomes imagination*. New York, NY: Basic; 2000. Print.

Ely JW, Osheroff JA, Ebell M. Analysis of questions asked by family doctors regarding patient care. *BMJ*. 1997; **319**: 358–61. Print.

Epstein RM. Mindful practice. *JAMA*. 1999; **292**(9): 833. Print.

Eraut M. Non-formal learning and tacit knowledge in professional work. *Br J Educ Psychol*. 2000; **70**(1): 113–36. Print.

Erickson HC, Tomlin EM, Price Swain MA. *Modeling and Role Modeling: a theory and paradigm for nursing.* Englewood Cliffs, NJ: Prentice-Hall; 1983. Print.

Ericsson KA. *The Cambridge Handbook of Expertise and Expert Performance.* Cambridge: Cambridge University Press; 2006. Print.

Ernst E. Obstacles to research in complementary and alternative medicine. *Med J Aust.* 2003; **179**(6): 279–80. Print.

Evans R. Releasing time to care: Productive Ward, survey results. *Nurs Times.* 2007; **10**(Suppl. 16): S6–9.

Eve R. *PUNs and DENs: discovering learning needs in general practice.* Oxford: Radcliffe Medical Press; 2003. Print.

Everett DL. *Don't Sleep, There Are Snakes: life and language in the Amazonian jungle.* New York: Pantheon; 2008. Print.

FearFighter. Panic & Phobia Treatment. CCBT Limited Healthcare online. Web. Available at: www.fearfighter.com

Festinger L. *A Theory of Cognitive Dissonance.* California: Stanford University Press; 1957. Print.

Figusch Z, editor. *From One-to-one Psychodrama to Large Group Socio-psychodrama: more writings from the arena of Brazilian psychodrama.* Figusch; 2009. Print.

Finke RA, Ward TB, Smith SM. *Creative Cognition: theory, research, and applications.* Cambridge, MA: MIT; 1996. Print.

Firth-Cozens J. Doctors, their wellbeing, and their stress. *BMJ.* 2003; **326**: 670–1. Print.

Flett G. York researcher finds that perfectionism can lead to imperfect health. *York's Daily Bulletin.* Toronto, Canada: York University; June 2004. Print.

Flood GD. *An Introduction to Hinduism.* New York, NY: Cambridge University Press; 1996. Print.

Flynn JR. *What Is Intelligence: beyond the Flynn Effect.* Expanded paperback ed. Cambridge: Cambridge University Press; 2009. Web. http://en.wikipedia.org/wiki/International_Standard_Book_Number

Foresight Project. *Mental Capital and Wellbeing: making the most of ourselves in the 21st century.* The Foresight Project. The Government Office for Science: London; 2008. Web.

Foucault M. *History of Madness.* London: Routledge; 2006. Print.

Fowler KA, Lilienfield SO, Patrick CJ. Detecting psychopathy from thin slices of behaviour. *Psychol Assess.* 2009; **21**: 68–78. Print.

Frackowiak RSJ, Ashburner JT, Penny WD *et al. Human Brain Function.* 2nd ed. San Diego, California: Academic Press; 2004. Print.

Frankel RM. From sentence to sequence: understanding the medical encounter through microinteractional analysis. *Discourse Processes.* 1984; **7**(2): 135–70. Print.

Fredrickson BL. The role of positive emotions in positive psychology: the broaden-and-build theory of positive emotions. *Am Psychol.* 2001; **56**(3): 218–26. Print.

Gabora L. The origin and evolution of culture and creativity. *Journal of Memetics.* 1997; **1**(1): n.p. Print.

Gardner, H. *Frames of Mind: The Theory of Multiple Intelligences.* 3rd ed. Basic Books, 2011. Print.

Gettier EL. Is justified true belief knowledge. *Analysis.* 1963. **23**: 121–3. Print.

Gibbs G. *Learning by Doing: a guide to teaching and learning methods.* [London]: FEU; 1988. Print.

Gilbert DT. *Stumbling on Happiness.* New York: Vintage; 2007. Print.

Gilbert E. *Eat, Pray, Love: one woman's search for everything.* New York: Penguin; 2006. Print.

Giles J. *No Self to Be Found: the search for personal identity.* Lanham: University of America; 1997. Print.

Gillon R. Medical ethics: 'four principles plus attention to scope'. *BMJ.* 1994; **309**: 184. Print.

Glaser BG, Strauss AS. *Awareness of Dying.* Chicago: Aldine Pub.; [1965]. Reprint 2005. Print.

GMC. *Disciplinary Decisions.* Rep. General Medical Council. Web. Available at: www.gmc-uk.org/concerns/hearings_and_decisions/fitness_to_practise_decisions.asp

GMC. *Good Medical Practice.* Rep. General Medical Council UK, 2006. Web. Available at: www.gmc-uk.org/guidance/good_medical_practice.asp

GMC. *Printable Documents.* Summer 2009. Web. Available at: www.gmc-uk.org/concerns/printable_documents.asp

Goldberg LR. The structure of phenotypic personality traits. *Am Psychol.* 1993; **48**: 26–34. Print.

GP Online. *A Registrar Survival Guide . . . setting up your consulting room.* GP Online. 2010. Web. Available at: www.gponline.com/Education/article/1037805/a-registrar-survival-guide-setting-consulting-room (accessed 4 November 2010).

GP Training Net. *Consultation Theory.* Web. Available at: http://gptraining.net (accessed 12 November 2011).

Grant J, Crawley J. *Transference and Projection: mirrors to the self.* Buckingham: Open University; 2002. Print.

Greene B. *The Elegant Universe: superstrings, hidden dimensions, and the quest for the ultimate theory.* London: Vintage; 2005. Print.

Greenhalgh T, Hurwitz B, editors. *Narrative Based Medicine: dialogue and discourse in clinical practice.* London: BMJ; 2002. Print.

Grimshaw GM, Stanton T. Tobacco cessation interventions for young people. *Cochrane Database Syst Rev.* 2006; **4**: CD003289. Print.

Haigh R. Modern milieux: therapeutic community solutions to acute ward problems. *The Psychiatrist.* 2002; **26**: 380–2. Print.

Haigh R. The quintessence of a therapeutic environment: five universal qualities. In: Campling P, Haigh R, editors. *Therapeutic Communities: past, present and future.* London: Jessica Kingsley; 1999. pp. 246–57. Print.

Hakeda YS. *Kukai: major works.* New York: Columbia University Press; 1972. Print.

Hall ET. *The Hidden Dimension.* Garden City, NY: Doubleday; 1966. Print.

Hammond DC. Review of the efficacy of clinical hypnosis with headaches and migraines. *IJCEH.* 2007; **55**(2): 207–19. Print.

Handy CB. *Gods of Management: the changing work of organizations.* New York: Oxford University Press; 1995. Print.

Handy CB. *Understanding Organisations.* Harmondsworth, Middlesex: Penguin; [1976] 1985. Print.

Hawking SW. *A Brief History of Time: from the big bang to black holes*. Toronto: Bantam; 1988. Print.

Health Foundation. *Evidence: helping people help themselves. A review of the evidence considering whether it is worthwhile to support self-management*. Health Foundation; May 2011. Web. Available at: www.health.org.uk/publications/evidence-helping-people-help-themselves

Health Talk Online. *Shared Decision Making*. Healthtalkonline. DOH. Web. Available at: www.healthtalkonline.org/Improving_health_care/shared_decision_making (accessed April 2011).

Hecht MA, LaFrance M. How (fast) can I help you? Tone of voice and telephone operator efficiency in interactions. *J Appl Soc Psychol*. 1995; **25**(23): 2086–98. Print.

Hélie S, Sun R. Incubation, insight, and creative problem solving: a unified theory and a connectionist model. *Psychol Rev*. 2010; **117**(3): 994–1024. Print.

Helman CG. Disease versus illness in general practice. *J R Coll Gen Pract*. 1981; **31**: 548–62. Print.

Hendrich A, Chow MP, Skierczynski BA, Lu Z. A 36-hospital time and motion study: how do medical-surgical nurses spend their time? *Perm J*. 2008; **12**(3): 25–34. Print.

Henning K, Ey S, Shaw D. Perfectionism, the impostor phenomenon and psychological adjustment in medical, dental, nursing and pharmacy students. *Med Educ*. 1998; **32**(5): 456–64. Print.

Hermans HJM, Gieser T. *Handbook of Dialogical Self Theory*. Cambridge: Cambridge University Press; 2011. Print.

Hermans HJM, Kempen HJG. *The Dialogical Self: meaning as movement*. San Diego: Academic; 1993. Print.

Heron J. A six-category intervention analysis. *Br J Guidance & Counselling*. 1976; **4**(2): 143–55. Print.

Herzberg F. *The Motivation to Work*. New York: Wiley; 1959. Print.

Hinduism Today. *Join the Hindu Renaissance*. Hinduism Today Magazine. Web. Available at: www.hinduismtoday.com (accessed 14 November 2011).

Hilbert D, Cohn-Vossen S. *Geometry and the Imagination*. 2nd ed. London: Chelsea Publishing Company; 1990. Print.

Hofstadter DR. *Gödel, Escher, Bach*. Harmondsworth: Penguin; 1980. Print.

Hume D. *A Treatise of Human Nature; being an attempt to introduce the experimental method of reasoning into moral subjects*. Cleveland: World Pub.; [1739] 1962. Print.

Hutton W. *The State We're In*. London: Jonathan Cape; 1995. Print.

Hymes J. editor. *The Child under Six*. London: Consortium; 1994. Print.

Ignatow D. *Against the Evidence: selected poems, 1934–1994*. [Middletown, Conn.]: Wesleyan University Press; 1993. Print.

Internet Encyclopedia of Philosophy. *Time*. Internet Encyclopedia of Philosophy. Web. Available at: www.iep.utm.edu/time (accessed 14 November 2011).

Isaksen SG, Treffinger DJ. *Creative Problem Solving: the basic course*. Buffalo, NY: Bearly; 1985. Print.

Isen A, Daubman KA, Nowicki GP. Positive affect facilitates creative problem solving. *J Pers Soc Psychol*. 1987; **52**(6): 1122–31. Print.

Ivancevich JM, Matteson MT. Stress and work: a managerial perspective. In: Quick JC, Bhagat RS, Dalton JE, Quick JD, editors. *Work Stress: health care systems in the workplace*. New York: Praeger; 1980. pp. 27–49. Print.

James W. *The Principles of Psychology*. Charleston, SC: BiblioLife; 2010. Print.

Juran JM, Gryna FM. *Juran's Quality Control Handbook*. New York: McGraw-Hill; 1988. Print.

Kabat-Zinn J. *Full Catastrophe Living: using the wisdom of your body and mind to face stress, pain, and illness*. New York, NY: Dell Pub., a Division of Bantam Doubleday Dell Pub. Group; 1991. Print.

Kahn RL, Byosiere P. Stress in organizations. In: Dunnette MD, Hough LM, editors. *Handbook of Industrial and Organizational Psychology, Vol. 3*. Palo Alto, CA: Consulting Psychologists Press; 1992. pp. 571–650. Print.

Kahneman D. *Thinking, Fast and Slow*. New York: Penguin; 2012. Print.

Kandel ER, Schwartz JM, Jessell TM. *Principles of Neural Science*. New York: McGraw-Hill, Health Professions Division; 2000. Print.

Kant I. *Groundwork for the Metaphysics of Morals*. New Haven: Yale University Press; 2002. Print.

Kaufman JC, Beghetto RA. Beyond big and little: the Four C Model of Creativity. *Rev Gen Psychology*. 2009; **13**: 1–12. Print.

Keating T. Centering Prayer. Web. Available at: www.centeringprayer.com (accessed 12 November 2011).

King LS. *Medical Thinking: a historical preface*. Princeton, NJ: Princeton University Press; 1982. Print.

Kleinke CL, Peterson TR, Rutledge TR. Effects of self-generated facial expressions on mood. *J Pers Soc Psychol*. 1998; **74**(1): 272–9. Print.

Kleinman A. *Patients and Healers in the Context of Culture: an exploration of the borderland between anthropology, medicine, and psychiatry*. Berkeley: University of California; 1980. Print.

Ko U. Ananda. *Beyond Self: 108 Korean Zen poems*. Berkeley, CA: Parallax; 1997. Print.

Koch R. *The Natural Laws of Business: applying the theories of Darwin, Einstein, and Newton to achieve business success*. New York: Currency/Doubleday; 2001. Print.

Koestler A. *The Ghost in the Machine*. London: Hutchinson; 1967. Print.

Kolb DA. *Experiential Learning: experience as the source of learning and development*. Englewood Cliffs, NJ: Prentice-Hall; 1984. Print.

Kornfield J. *Buddha's Little Instruction Book*. London: Rider & Co; 1996. Print.

Kotter JP. *Leading Change*. Boston, MA: Harvard Business School; 1996. Print.

Kumar M. *Quantum: Einstein, Bohr, and the great debate about the nature of reality*. New York: W.W. Norton; 2009. Print.

Kurtz SM, Silverman J, Draper J. *Teaching and Learning Communication Skills in Medicine*. Oxford: Radcliffe Publishing; 2005. Print.

Lalor D. *Creating a Therapeutic Environment. Counselling in Perth, Western Australia*. Cottesloe Counselling Centre. Web. Available at: www.cottesloecounselling.com.au (accessed 24 October 2011).

Lazarus RS, Folkman S. *Stress, Appraisal, and Coping*. New York: Springer; 1984.

Launer J. *Narrative-based Primary Care: a practical guide*. Oxford: Radcliffe Medical Press; 2002. Print.

Légaré F, Ratté S, Stacey D, *et al*. Interventions for improving the adoption of shared decision making by healthcare professionals. *Cochrane Database Syst Rev*. 2011; **10**: CD001431. Web.

Lehrer J. *Imagine: how creativity works*. Edinburgh: Canongate; 2012. Print.

Levensky E, Forcehimes A, Beitz K. Motivational interviewing: an evidence-based approach to counseling helps patients follow treatment recommendations. *Am J Nurs*. 2007; **107**(10): 50–8. Print.

Lewin S, Skea Z, Entwistle V, *et al*. Effects of interventions to promote a patient-centred approach in clinical consultations. *Cochrane Database Syst Rev*. 2001; **4**: CD00326. Web.

Lewin SA, Skea Z, Entwistle VA, *et al*. Interventions for providers to promote a patient-centred approach in clinical consultations. *Cochrane Database Syst Rev*. 2012; **12**: CD003267. Print.

Linehan M. *Cognitive Behavioural Treatment of Borderline Personality Disorder*. London: Guildford; 1993. Print.

Linn LS, Yager J, Cope D, Leake B. Health status, job satisfaction, job stress, and life satisfaction among academic and clinical faculty. *JAMA*. 1985; **254**(19): 2775–82. Print.

Living Life to the Full. *Free Online Skills Course*. Living Life to the Full. Web. Available at: www.llttf.com (accessed 28 October 2011).

Locke J, Bassett T, Holt E. *An Essay Concerning Humane Understanding: in four books*. London: Printed by Eliz. Holt for Thomas Basset; 1690. Print.

Mackenzie RA. *The Time Trap*. New York: AMACOM; 1972. Print.

Maslach C, Schaufeli W, Leiter M. Job burnout. *Annu Rev Psychol*. 2001; **52**: 397–422. Web.

Maslow AH. A theory of human motivation. *Psychol Rev*. 1943; **50**(4): 370–96. Print.

Maslow AH. *The Farther Reaches of Human Nature*. New York: Penguin; 1976. Print.

May R. *The Courage to Create*. London: Collins; 1976. Print.

McCambridge J. Motivational interviewing is equivalent to more intensive treatment, superior to placebo, and will be tested more widely. *Evidence-Based Mental Health*. 2004. **7**(2): 52. Print.

McKinlay JB, Potter DA, Feldman DA. Non-medical influences on medical decision-making. *Soc Sci Med*. 1996; **42**(5): 769–76. Print.

McQuaid JR, Carmona PE. *Peaceful Mind: using mindfulness and cognitive behavioral psychology to overcome depression*. Oakland, CA: New Harbinger; 2004. Print.

McVicar A. Workplace stress in nursing: a literature review. *J Adv Nurs*. 2003; **44**(6): 633–42. Print.

Melville A. Job satisfaction in general practice: implications for prescribing. *Soc Sci Med. Part A: Medical Psychology & Medical Sociology*. 1980; **14**(6): 495–9. Print.

Mitchley SE. The medical interview: the three-function approach. *Postgrad Med J*. 1992; **68**(799): 397–8. Print.

MoodGYM. Welcome. Web. Available at: www.moodgym.anu.edu.au (accessed 28 October 2011).

Moran P. *Antisocial Personality Disorder*. London: Gaskell; 1999. Print.

Morrison T. *Staff Supervision in Social Care: making a real difference for staff and service users*. Brighton: Pavilion; 2005. Print.

National Institute for Health and Care Excellence. *Anxiety: management of anxiety (panic disorder, with or without agoraphobia, and generalised anxiety disorder) in adults in primary, secondary and community care*. NICE. March 2011. Web. Available at: http://guidance.nice.org.uk/CG22

National Institute for Health and Care Excellence. *Brief Interventions and Referral for Smoking Cessation in Primary Care and Other Settings*. NICE. 2006. Web. Available at: www.nice.org.uk/nicemedia/pdf/SMOKING-ALS2_FINAL.pdf

National Institute for Health and Care Excellence. *Cognitive Behavioural Therapy for the Management of Common Mental Health Problems*. NICE. December 2010. Web. Available at: www.nice.org.uk/usingguidance/commissioningguides/cognitivebehavioural therapyservice/cbt.jsp

National Institute for Health and Care Excellence. *Computerised Cognitive Behaviour Therapy for Depression and Anxiety: review of Technology Appraisal 51*. NICE. February 2006. Web. Available at: www.nice.org.uk/nicemedia/pdf/TA097guidance.pdf

Neighbour R. *The Inner Consultation: how to develop an effective and intuitive consulting style*. Lancaster: MTP; 1987. Print.

NHS Centre for Reviews. *Effectiveness Matters: counselling in primary care*. 2001; **5**(2): n.p. Print.

NHS Direct. *Decision Aids*. NHS Direct. Web. Available at: www.nhsdirect.nhs.uk/decisionaids.

NHS Institute for Innovation and Improvement. *Releasing Time to Care: the productive ward*. 2007. Available at: www.institute.nhs.uk/quality_and_value/productivity_series/productive_ward.html.

Noonuccal, Oodgeroo. *My People*. 3rd ed. Milton, QA: The Jacaranda Press; 1990. Print.

Ogedegbe G. Labeling and hypertension: it is time to intervene on its negative consequences. *Hypertension*. 2010; **56**(3): 344–5. Print.

O'Hara LA. Creativity and intelligence. In: Sternberg RJ, editor. *Handbook of Creativity*. Cambridge University Press; 1999. Print.

Open Door Coaching. *Job Satisfaction Inventory*. Open Door Coaching. Web. Available at: www.opendoorcoaching.com/PDF%20files/Job%20Satisfaction%20Inventory.PDF (accessed 24 October 2011).

Orwell G. *Nineteen Eighty-four, a novel*. New York: Harcourt, Brace; 1949. Print.

'Overcoming' series. Constable & Robinson Publishers. Web. Available at: www.overcoming.co.uk

Paice E, Moss F. How important are role models in making good doctors. *BMJ*. 2002; **325**: 707. Print.

Patient.co.uk. *Significant Event Analysis*. Health Information and Advice, Medicines Guide, Patient.co.uk. Web. Available at: http://patient.co.uk (accessed 24 October 2011).

Patrick CJ, Craig KD, Prkachin KM. Observer judgments of acute pain: facial action determinants. *J Pers Soc Psych*. 1986; **50**(6): 1291–8. Print.

Pendleton D, Schofield T, Tate P, Havelock P. *The Consultation: an approach to learning and teaching*. Oxford: Oxford University Press; 1984. Print.

Penrose R. *The Emperor's New Mind: concerning computers, minds, and the laws of physics*. Oxford: Oxford University Press; 1989. Print.

Pepler D J. Play and divergent thinking. In: Pepler DJ, Rubin KH. *The Play of Children: current theory and research*. Basel; New York: Karger; 1982. Print.

Pepler DJ, Rubin KH, editors. *The Play of Children: current theory and research*. Basel; New York: Karger; 1982. Print.

Prkachin KM. Dissociating spontaneous and deliberate expressions of pain: signal detection analyses. *Pain*. 1992; **51**(1): 57–65. Print.

Prochaska JO, DiClemente CC. *The Transtheoretical Approach: crossing traditional boundaries of therapy*. Malabar, Florida: R. E. Krieger; 1994. Print.

Proshansky H. The field of environmental psychology. *Handbook of Environmental Psychology*. New York: Wiley; 1987. Print.

Proshansky H, Fabian A, Kaminoff R. Place-identity: physical world socialization of the self. *J Environ Psychol*. 1983; **3**(1): 57–83. Print.

Quakers. *Quaker Faith & Practice: the book of Christian discipline of the yearly meeting of the Religious Society of Friends (Quakers) in Britain*. London: Yearly Meeting of the Religious Society of Friends (Quakers) in Britain; 2009. Print.

Reuler JB, Nardone DA. Role modeling in medical education. *West J Med*. 1994; **160**(4): 335–7. Print.

Rolfe G, Freshwater D, Jasper M. *Critical Reflection for Nursing and the Helping Professions: a user's guide*. Houndmills, Basingstoke, Hampshire: Palgrave; 2001. Print.

Rossman J. *Industrial Creativity; the psychology of the inventor*. New Hyde Park, NY: University; 1964. Print.

Roter DL, Frankel RM, Hall JA, Sluyter D. The expression of emotion through nonverbal behavior in medical visits. Mechanisms and outcomes. *J Gen Intern Med*. 2006; **21**(Suppl. 1): S28–34. Print.

Sackett DL, Rosenberg WM, Gray JA, *et al*. Evidence based medicine: what it is and what it isn't. *BMJ*. 1996; **312**: 71–2. Print.

Sandman, L, Munthe C. Shared decision making, paternalism and patient choice. *Health Care Anal*. 2010; **18**(1): 60–84. Print.

Schegloff EA, Jefferson G, Sacks H. The preference for self-correction in the organization of repair in conversation. *Language*. 1977; **53**: 361–82. Print.

Schön DA. *The Reflective Practitioner: how professionals think in action*. Aldershot: Ashgate; [1983] 2002. Print.

Schwarz, B. *The Paradox of Choice: why more is less*. HarperCollins; New edition; 2005. Print.

Searle JR. *Mind: a brief introduction*. Oxford: Oxford University Press; 2004. Print.

Segal Z, Williams JM, Teasdale J. *Mindfulness-Based Cognitive Therapy for Depression: a new approach to preventing relapse*. New York: Guildford; 2001. Print.

Seligman MEP. *Authentic Happiness: using the new positive psychology to realize your potential for lasting fulfillment*. New York: Free; 2002. Print.

Sharot T, De Martino B, Dolan RJ. Neural activity predicts attitude change in cognitive dissonance. *Nature Neuroscience*. 2009; **29**(12): 3760–5. Print.

Silverman J, Kurtz SM, Draper J. *Skills for Communicating with Patients*. 3rd ed. London: Radcliffe Publishing; 2013. Print.

Simon HA. The mind's eye in chess. In: Chase WG, editor. *Visual Information Processing.* New York: Academic; 1973. Print.

Simon P, Garfunkel A. *The Sounds of Silence.* Columbia, released 1965. CD.

Simonton DK. Creativity, leadership, and chance. In: Sternberg RJ, editor. *The Nature of Creativity.* Cambridge: Cambridge University Press; 1988. Print.

Smith HW. *The 10 Natural Laws of Successful Time and Life Management: proven strategies for increased productivity and inner peace.* New York, NY: Warner; 2003. Print.

Snyder CR, Lopez SJ, editors. *Handbook of Positive Psychology.* Oxford: Oxford University Press; 2009. Print.

Soria R, Legido A, Escolano C. A randomised controlled trial of motivational interviewing for smoking cessation. *Br J Gen Pract.* 2006; **1**(56): 531. Print.

Sowa JF. 'Representing knowledge soup in language and logic'. Available online at: www. jfsowa.com/talks/souprepr.htm

Sternberg RJ. *Beyond IQ: A Triarchic Theory of Intelligence.* Cambridge: Cambridge University Press; 1985.

Stewart I, Joines V. *TA Today: a new introduction to transactional analysis.* Nottingham: Lifespace Pub.; 1987. Print.

Stewart M, Roter D. *Communicating with Medical Patients.* Newbury Park: Sage Publications; 1989. Print.

Stiglitz JE, Sen A, Fitoussi J-P. *Report by the Commission on the Measurement of Economic Performance and Social Progress.* Paris: Commission; 2009. Print.

Stott NC, Davis RH. The exceptional potential in each primary care consultation. *J R Coll Gen Pract.* 1979; **29**: 201–5. Print.

Suzuki DT. *Essays in Zen Buddhism, third series.* London: Published for the Buddhist Society by Rider; 1958. Print.

Suzuki S, Dixon T. *Zen Mind, Beginner's Mind.* New York: Walker/Weatherhill; 1970. Print.

Tarski A. *Logic, Semantics, Metamathematics; papers from 1923 to 1938.* Oxford: Clarendon; 1956. Print.

Taylor D, Bury M. Chronic illness, expert patients and care transition. *Sociology of Health & Illness.* 2007; **29**(1): 27–45. Print.

Tellegen A, Lykken DT, Bouchard TJ, *et al.* Personality similarity in twins reared apart and together. *J Pers Soc Psychol.* 1988; **54**(6): 1031–9. Print.

Thich Nhat Hanh, Mobi Ho, Vo-Dinh Mai. *Miracle of Mindfulness: an introduction.* Boston: Beacon; 1975. Print.

Top Nursing Colleges. *Nursing Theories and Sub-theories.* Top Nursing Colleges. Web. Available at: www.topnursingcolleges.com/nur/nursing-theories-and-sub-theories. html (accessed 12 November 2011).

Tsao L. How much do we know about the importance of play in child development. *Childhood Educ.* Summer 2002. Findarticles.com. Web. Available at: http://findarticles. com/p/articles/mi_qa3614/is_200207/ai_n9147500

Tuckett D, Boulton M, Olson C, Williams A. *Meetings between Experts: an approach to sharing ideas in medical consultations.* London: Tavistock, 1985. Print.

Ubel PA, Angott AM, Zikmund-Fischer BJ. Physicians recommend different treatment for patients than they would choose for themselves. *Arch Intern Med.* 2011; **171**(18): 630–4. Print.

Ulrich RS. How design impacts wellness. *Healthc Forum J.* 1992; **35**(5): 20–5. Print.

Upton J. *Comments.* FearFighter for Panic and Anxiety. Web. Available at: www.fear fighter.com (accessed 28 October 2011).

US National Cancer Institute. *Cancer Screening Overview (PDQ®).* US National Cancer Institute. Web. Available at: www.cancer.gov/cancertopics/pdq/screening/overview/HealthProfessional/page1 (accessed 24 October 2011).

Van Ham I, Verhoeven A, Groenier K, Groothoff J and De Haan J. Job satisfaction among general practitioners: A systematic literature review. *Eur J Gen Pract.* 2006, **12**(4): 174–80. (doi:10.1080/13814780600994376)

Van Veen V, Krug MK, Scooler JW, Carter CS. Neural activity predicts attitude change in cognitive dissonance. *Nature Neuroscience.* 2009; **12**(11): 1469–74. Print.

Vandervert L, Schimpf P, Liu H. How working memory and the cerebellum collaborate to produce creativity and innovation. *Creativity Res J.* 2007; **19**(1): 1–18. Print.

Various. Evidence based practice in clinical hypnosis. *IJCEH.* 2007; **55**(2): n.p. Print.

Walker L. *Consulting with NLP: Neuro-linguistic Programming in the medical consultation.* Oxford: Radcliffe Medical Press; 2002. Print.

Wallas G. *The Art of Thought.* New York: Harcourt, Brace; 1926. Print.

Warren KS. *Coping with the Biomedical Literature: a primer for the scientist and the clinician.* New York, NY: Praeger; 1981. Print.

Waskett C. An integrated approach to introducing and maintaining supervision: the 4S Model. *Nurs Times.* 2009; **105**(17): 24–6. Print.

Weisberg RW. *Creativity: beyond the myth of genius.* New York: W.H. Freeman; 1993. Print.

West C. Against our will: male interruptions of females in cross-sex conversation. *Annals of the New York Academy of Sciences.* 1979 (Language, Sex); **327**(1): 81–96. Print.

White M. *Maps of Narrative Practice.* New York: W.W. Norton & Co; 2007. Print.

White M, Epston D. *Narrative Means to Therapeutic Ends.* New York: Norton; 1990. Print.

Wilber K. *A Brief History of Everything.* Boston, MA: Shambhala; 2007. Print.

Wilber K. An integral theory of consciousness. *J Consciousness Stud.* 1997; **4**(1): 71–92. Print.

Williams CJ, Garland A. Cognitive-behavioural therapy assessment model for use in clinical practice. *Adv Psych Treat.* 2002; **8**: 172–79. Print.

Williams ES, Konrad TR. Physician, practice, and patient characteristics related to primary care physician physical and mental health: results from the Physician Worklife Study. *Health Services Res.* 2002; **37**(1): 119–41. Print.

Williams ES, Konrad TR, Scheckler WE, *et al.* Understanding physicians' intentions to withdraw from practice: the role of job satisfaction, job stress, mental and physical health. *Health Care Manage Rev.* 2010; **35**(2): 105–15. Web.

Wilson PM, Kendall S, Brooks F. The Expert Patients Programme: a paradox of patient empowerment and medical dominance. *Health & Social Care in the Community.* 2007; **15**(5): 426–38. Web.

Yovel G, Kanwisher N. Face perception: domain specific, not process specific. *Neuron.* 2004; **44**(5): 889–98. Print.

Zhong E, Kenward K, Sheets V, *et al.* Probation and recidivism: remediation among disciplined nurses in six states. *Am J Nurs.* 2009; **109**(3): 48–57. Print.

CPD with Radcliffe

You can now use a selection of our books to achieve CPD (Continuing Professional Development) points through directed reading.

We provide a free online form and downloadable certificate for your appraisal portfolio. Look for the CPD logo and register with us at: www.radcliffehealth.com/cpd

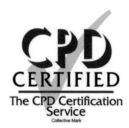